"*The Trauma-Informed Workbook for Addiction* is a co[mprehensive guide to] recovery. Darla Belflower masterfully connects the [...] offering practical tools and guidance. This workbook [empowers individuals to heal with know]edge, self-awareness, and actionable skills. It is a must-read for those on the path to recovery and the professionals who support them."

—**Erin Fraser, LCSW**, executive director of Benilde Hall

"Darla Belflower has created something special for those that work in the substance use field or have had their own journey with substance use. Using her professional and personal experience, strength, and hope, she has created material so useful for those inflicted with trauma and substance use that recognizes and acknowledges how these almost always go hand and hand."

—**Shayna Parker, LCSW**, adult/adolescent mental health/trauma therapist, and alumni of Saint Louis University

"*The Trauma-Informed Workbook for Addiction* is truly inspiring, impactful, and amazing! The workbook is broken down into simple yet descriptive terminology, providing real-life examples, and with direct application practices to your own life. I wish I would have had a workbook like this when I began my own recovery journey four years ago. Darla Belflower's workbook comes from a place of experience rooted in both personal depth and professional wisdom."

—**Nicole Arnsmeyer, MSEd, CPS**, coordinator/educator for GED/HiSET program; and recovery coordinator at Healing House, Inc

"Darla Belflower's *The Trauma-Informed Workbook for Addiction* is a powerful, compassionate resource that blends evidence-based practices with deep insight into the roots of substance use and trauma. As an LCSW and former therapist, I appreciate the practical tools and thoughtful structure that guide readers toward healing and lasting recovery. This workbook is an essential companion for anyone seeking to understand their trauma, build resilience, and reclaim their life."

—**David Stoecker, LCSW, CPS, HRS**, executive director of Better Life in Recovery, and cofounder of Springfield Recovery Community Center

"Comprehensive, powerful, and grounded in current best practices, *The Trauma-Informed Workbook for Addiction* offers a compassionate approach to healing, and is a relevant and indispensable tool for navigating the journey of recovery in modern times. This workbook is not just helpful for those on their recovery journey, but for their loved ones and professionals alike."

—**James Glenn, MSW**, associate administrator of business strategies at University Health Behavioral Health, and codirector of the Mid-America Addiction Technology Transfer Center (ATTC)

"Darla Belflower brings the heart of a seasoned clinician and the understanding of someone who truly walks alongside those in recovery. *The Trauma-Informed Workbook for Addiction* offers practical, compassionate tools for healing, making it an essential guide for anyone navigating the intersection of trauma and substance use."

—**Kenneth A. Vick, LAC, CPS**, executive director of Avalon Wellness & Recovery, and author of *Recovery Leadership*

The Trauma-Informed Workbook for Addiction

Evidence-Based Skills to Heal the Pain at the Root of
Your Substance Use and Build Resilience for Lasting Recovery

DARLA BELFLOWER, LCSW

New Harbinger Publications, Inc.

Publisher's Note

This publication is designed to provide accurate and authoritative information in regard to the subject matter covered. It is sold with the understanding that the publisher is not engaged in rendering psychological, financial, legal, or other professional services. If expert assistance or counseling is needed, the services of a competent professional should be sought.

NEW HARBINGER PUBLICATIONS is a registered trademark of New Harbinger Publications, Inc.

New Harbinger Publications is an employee-owned company.

Copyright © 2025 by Darla Belflower
    New Harbinger Publications, Inc.
    5720 Shattuck Avenue
    Oakland, CA 94609
    www.newharbinger.com

All Rights Reserved

Cover design by Amy Daniel

Acquired by Jess O'Brien

Edited by Joyce Wu

Library of Congress Cataloging-in-Publication Data on file

Printed in the United States of America

27	26	25								
10	9	8	7	6	5	4	3	2	1	First Printing

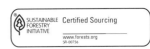

This workbook is dedicated to everyone who makes recovery possible, those who have faced the challenges of substance use disorder and trauma, and those whose support makes those challenges a little easier to bear.

To the families and friends who support their loved ones through the hardest of times, your support is a big part of their recovery and success. That support and compassion are invaluable. Please remember to take care of yourselves in your own journey of healing, because you cannot support someone else if you are not well.

To the healthcare professionals, counselors, therapists, case managers, and peer support workers who have dedicated themselves to helping others find their way to healing, thank you for your commitment and care. So many of us would not have been able to reach recovery without the support of professionals such as you. May you continue to carry the hope for others, until they can carry it for themselves.

Finally, and most importantly, this workbook is dedicated to *you*. Entering recovery is not an easy choice. Rather, it is a choice that takes radical bravery. As you work to heal, may this workbook be a source of hope, strength, and guidance, no matter what path you choose to take.

Together, we acknowledge the pain of the past, embrace the strength of the present, and look forward to the possibilities of the future.

With deepest respect and admiration,

Darla

Contents

	Foreword	vii
	Introduction	1
Chapter 1	What Is Substance Use Disorder?	3
Chapter 2	What Is Trauma?	19
Chapter 3	The Connection Between Trauma and Substance Use Disorder	33
Chapter 4	Embarking on the Road to Recovery	49
Chapter 5	Forgiveness	65
Chapter 6	Self-Esteem	81
Chapter 7	Relationships	97
Chapter 8	Meditation: The Gift of Inner Listening	113
Chapter 9	Gratitude	119
Chapter 10	Recovery Planning	135
	Conclusion: Embracing the Journey of Recovery	151
	Acknowledgments	154
	Resources	155
	References	160

Foreword

I began providing recovery housing in 2003 as the next step of my own recovery from addiction. In those early years, I did not understand the impact of trauma on myself or the people that I served. I knew that I had been scarred by homelessness, abuse, sexual assault, and prostitution, but I did not use the word "trauma" to describe my experiences. I believed that somehow everything that happened to me was my fault. I had a speech impediment and was a chubby kid and so I grew up with low self-esteem. I started drinking to make those feelings of being the chubby kid who talked funny go away. Alcohol transformed me into the person I had always wanted to be: funny, popular and cute. I felt like I fit in.

At fifteen, I was in a car accident, while out with friends who were using and drinking. I had serious injuries. And for the next year, I was in a metal body cast, taking several pain medications—often over-taking them. My drinking continued during this time, even while I took these medications. I was not going to let being in a body cast stop me from partying and so I continued to go out and drink. Just before my sixteenth birthday, I was assaulted while in that body cast. I could not fight back. The pain and shame that I felt was only made bearable by using more pain medication and drinking. When the body cast was finally removed, I should have felt free—but once it was removed, so were my pain medications. I experienced my first delirium tremens, from which I could only get relief by using more pills and drinking.

I would like to say that my experience was unique to me and that other people who have addictions do not experience the pain and trauma that I have. What I have found in my work with others is that trauma and addiction go hand in hand. A few years back, I was doing a group for the women who live in my recovery houses. A young lady had come in the day before, and she was traumatized because she had been sexually assaulted shortly before coming in. She was so sad, almost like all her hope was gone. The room had maybe a hundred women in it, and I asked how many had experienced this type of assault. Even I was surprised when all but one of those women raised their hand.

In working with my male participants, they too have experienced trauma and the dysfunction that is left behind. What I see over and over at Healing House is that when our participants do not deal with their trauma, they continue to look for ways to relieve the pain they have and continue to have. If a person does not go back to using substances, they may have other coping strategies like smoking, overeating, sex, or gambling. It is not until they look at that pain and find new ways to deal with it that they really recover. Trauma bends our ability to see what's the cause of our pain. Finding new skills is the first step to finding purpose, and finding purpose leads to doing esteem able acts, which leads to higher self-esteem.

This workbook on treating your trauma as a path to your healing from addiction is a valuable tool to help anyone work on those new coping strategies and deal with life instead of dealing with addiction. This workbook has many different tools to help you move through the process. So much more is known now about how trauma or traumatic events can affect someone, much more than when I first entered my own recovery almost thirty years ago. I am excited to be able to place this workbook in our participants' hands to use while they work their way through their early recovery.

—Bobbi Jo Reed
Founder and CEO, Healing House Kansas City
Certified peer specialist and harm reduction specialist

Introduction

When I started working in the field of substance use disorder, it was a very different world than it is today. There was a belief that if a person had a substance use disorder and a mental health disorder, including post-traumatic stress disorder (PTSD), the person needed to get one treated before the other could be treated. This was known as sequential treatment. The problem with this was that no providers looked at both disorders—a person had to go to different agencies for treatment. The other problem was that there was no consensus about the "right" order of sequential treatment. If a person went to an organization that treated substance use disorder and had a mental health disorder like PTSD, they were often told that they needed to go to someplace else to get treatment for the PTSD before they could get treatment for their substance use disorder. So the person would drive across town to get treatment for their PTSD only to be told they needed treatment for their substance use first. This would cause a great number of folks to give up all together.

As more research has been done, we know that having both a substance use disorder and either PTSD or some of the symptoms of it as a result of trauma is the rule rather than the exception. In fact, in my practice I find that almost everyone I see for substance use disorder also has experienced trauma. Trauma is a risk factor for substance use and substance use is also a risk factor for trauma. It is important to understand that the two are linked and one can influence the other. These experiences of trauma can shape how we see and respond to the world. Experiencing trauma can create a feeling of not being safe, fear, and doubt in our ability to cope with situations that would otherwise not be an issue.

As you move through this workbook, it is my hope that you will have a better understanding of how your relationship with substances and the trauma you have experienced are influencing the way you move through your life, and how one may create difficulty in looking at and coping with the other. It is by looking at both that true healing and movement forward can occur.

I entered my own recovery many years ago. Throughout this workbook, I will share some of my own stories and what I've learned. For example, it has been my experience that there are certain things that enhance getting the most from a life in recovery. Some of these include forgiveness of the past, increasing your self-esteem, how you show up for the relationships you are in, and how meditation, gratitude, and recovery planning form the foundation of a solid plan for recovery.

It is my hope, as you work your way through this workbook, that it is not only helpful helpful for you now but that you can use it as a tool well into your future as you navigate your recovery journey. I encourage you to not race through the workbook, but to take your time and to really think about the exercises that are presented. At the same time, I know that I am often hard on myself and want to get things right or perfect the first time. Give yourself permission to be human and take it easy on yourself. We are often our own worst critics. I would like you to gain the benefit of the exercises and not focus on doing them perfectly.

If no one has told you, you are a miracle. The fact that you are here, reading this, working on some issues that may not be pleasant to address, says a lot about who you are and who you want to be. My hope for you is that you will gain some knowledge about yourself and find and create some tools that will help you as you work toward your goals.

Chapter 1

What Is Substance Use Disorder?

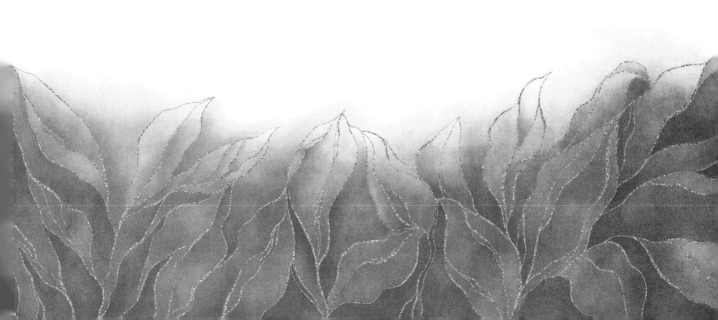

Substance use disorder is a condition of ongoing use of drugs and/or alcohol despite negative consequences. Substance use disorder is a disease of the brain. The substances that are used change the brain's structure and function, leading to cravings for more substances (Volkow and Morales 2015). Substance use disorder can cause significant impairment in various areas of a person's life. Some of the areas that are affected are work, school, relationships, finances, spirituality, and overall health. It can also lead to legal and financial problems, as well as an increased risk of overdose and other serious health complications. Statistics on the number of people in America with a substance use disorder vary based on when and how those numbers are collected. As a provider of substance use disorder services, I saw an increase in the number of people seeking help during the start of the COVID-19 pandemic in 2020, when many people were isolated—which points to the influences that society and our environments can also have on our substance use.

Substance use disorder was defined as a disease in 1956 by the American Medical Association and the American Society of Addiction Medicine. Recognizing substance use disorder as a disease, as opposed to a choice, has reduced the stigma often associated with it. Some people still believe substance use disorder is not a disease, as they see someone's substance use as a choice to consume substances. While the initial decision to use drugs or alcohol may be voluntary, substance use disorder is a chronic and complex disease that changes the brain's chemistry and circuitry, leading to a loss of control over one's behavior.

It is important to recognize that personal choice is not the determining factor in whether something is a disease. For instance, heart disease, diabetes, and some types of cancer can be influenced by personal choices like diet, exercise, and sun exposure. However, they are classified as diseases because of the physical changes that occur in the body due to those choices. Similarly, medical associations recognize substance use disorder as a disease based on the changes it causes in the brain.

The Brain and Substance Use Disorder

Continued use of substances can have an impact on the brain and the way it functions. Repeated substance misuse can cause changes in the way your brain works. Let's take caffeine, for example. Many of us drink coffee in the morning and it helps us start our day. When we drink it, we feel more awake and it brings us pleasure. That is because our brain releases dopamine, which causes us to feel good. But what happens when we drink coffee or other caffeinated beverages all day, in high amounts, over a period of time? Our brain becomes accustomed to those high levels of dopamine, and when we take it away, we feel some real physical consequences. We become tired, our heads hurt, and we may even be irritable. It becomes hard to enjoy ourselves when we are feeling this way. The same thing is true when we use other substances. As the substance use continues, it can interfere with the brain's reward system, making it difficult for individuals to experience pleasure from normal activities. Over time, this can lead to compulsive substance-seeking behavior to prevent us from feeling the negative impacts of discontinued use.

Substance use also interferes with parts of the brain responsible for cognitive function, leading to memory problems, difficulty with decision making, and reduced impulse control. The impact ongoing substance use can have on the brain appears to be long lasting. The younger a person is when they start using substances, the more likely they are to develop a substance use disorder later in life. Kids who use substances before the age of fourteen are four times more likely to develop a substance use disorder later in life (National Institute on Drug Abuse 2020).

If you've picked up this workbook, it's likely that you already know that you have both a substance use disorder and a history of trauma. However, some of you may be unsure if your substance use qualifies as substance misuse or a substance use disorder. It's common to not know. Let's take a look at your use more closely so that you can fully understand where you are.

Substance Use Screening

A screening is a brief set of questions used to determine if a more in-depth assessment is needed. An assessment is a more detailed process of gathering detailed information about a person's substance use. The following simple screening tool is used by many physicians and therapists to identify if alcohol use is a problem, but it can be used for other substances as well.

The acronym CAGE (Ewing 1984) represents the focus of the questions:

C: Cutting down—whether you've tried to cut down on your use

A: Annoyance of criticism—whether others annoy you with their criticism of your use

G: Guilty feeling—assessing your feelings about your use

E: Eye-opener—whether your dependency is such that you need substances to function

CAGE Screening

Circle the answer that best fits your experience with substances:

1. Have you ever felt you should cut down on your drinking or drug use? **Yes** or **No**

2. Have people annoyed you by criticizing your drinking or drug use? **Yes** or **No**

3. Have you ever felt guilty about your drinking or drug use? **Yes** or **No**

4. Have you ever had a drink or used drugs first thing in the morning to steady your nerves or to get rid of a hangover (eye-opener)? **Yes** or **No**

Scoring:

Count 0 for "no" and 1 for "yes" answers.

A total score of 2 or greater is considered significant.

Of course, CAGE is a simple screening tool. Many other factors are considered when looking at a formal diagnosis of substance use disorder. Below is the list of indicators that your substance use may be a problem. Check off any of the items that have been problems for you:

☐ You have used more substances (drugs or alcohol) than you intended to.

☐ You have wanted to stop using, but have not been able to cut down or stop.

☐ Time is spent recovering from using too much of the substance the day before.

☐ You think about using.

☐ Your substance use has caused problems between you and the people you love.

☐ You don't care as much about your work or friends.

☐ You have done dangerous things when using, like drinking and driving.

☐ You have to drink or use more substances to get the feeling you want.

☐ You go into withdrawal when you don't use.

How many did you check? The greater the number, the more likely it is that you have an unhealthy relationship with substances.

Ultimately, the most severe symptom of substance use disorder is the development of withdrawal symptoms, which are relieved only by taking more of the substance. If you find yourself in this situation, you should seek medical care. Withdrawal from certain substances like alcohol and benzodiazepines (Xanax, Librium, Tranxene, Valium, Lorazepam, Ativan, and Klonopin) can be life threatening and should be monitored closely.

You may want to journal about your experience below. What experiences have you had that indicate you're struggling with a substance use disorder? How have they affected your life?

Risk Factors

A risk factor is anything that increases the likelihood of something happening. A "because of this, that may happen," if you will. An example of this is that smoking cigarettes is a risk factor for developing lung cancer. Some mental health conditions increase the likelihood of developing problematic substance use. Having a diagnosis of PTSD increases the risk of developing a substance use disorder—people with PTSD use substances at a higher rate than those without a trauma history (Marschall 2023). The term "self-medication" refers to using substances as a way to numb or cope with the challenges of a mental health disorder, including the impact of trauma. Unfortunately, substance use can worsen the symptoms of the mental health condition, leading to a cycle of worsening symptoms of the trauma followed by an increase in the substance use.

One type of risk factor for developing a substance use disorder is heredity, or genetic predisposition. That is, if your parents engaged in problematic substance use, it can make it more likely that you will too. Studies have found that children of parents with substance use disorder are more likely to develop the disorder themselves, even if raised in a different environment. Ultimately, genetics accounts for about 50 percent of the risk for developing a substance use disorder (NIDA 2018).

Environment can be another risk for developing substance use disorder and can include many different influences—from family and friends to economic status and general quality of life. Things like peer pressure, physical and sexual abuse, early exposure to drugs, stress, and parental guidance can increase risks.

Social determinants of health describe certain factors in the conditions in which people are born, live, learn, and work that affect how well they're able to thrive. These factors include access to fresh and healthy food, safe housing, healthcare, transportation, safe neighborhoods, and technology. If you do not have regular, reliable access to these things, it can put you at risk for a wide range of health concerns, including substance use disorders (WHO n.d.).

Peer pressure—being around people who use substances and encourage you, directly or indirectly, to use—can contribute to substance use disorder, especially among teens who may feel pressure to fit in with their friends. Young people, however, are not the only ones susceptible to the pressures of substance use. In some families, drinking and drug use are common and an expected part of many social events, including family gatherings, weddings, sporting events, and funerals. All of this can normalize substance misuse.

Lack of social support and isolation is also be a risk factor when it comes to substance use. Feelings of loneliness are sometimes temporarily relieved by using a substance. For example, at the height of the COVID-19 pandemic, 13 percent of adults in America reported an increase in their substance use as a way to cope with the stress or emotions of isolation (Abramson 2021). Overdoses also increased during the pandemic as we all faced social isolation (Tanz et al. 2022).

Trauma and the way that we process it, or don't process it, is perhaps one of the strongest factors of a substance use disorder, whether experienced in childhood or later in life. Trauma can be defined as exposure to an incident or a series of emotionally disturbing or life-threatening events, which goes on to have lasting adverse effects on your functioning and well-being. Sometimes, when we're dealing with the intense feelings and memories that trauma can leave us with, substance use becomes the only coping mechanism we feel we have. Ultimately, the inability to appropriately deal with our emotions is often seen as the core issue of substance use disorder.

Have you ever considered your own risk factors for substance use disorder? As you look at the factors below, check the boxes that apply to you:

- ☐ **Genetic predisposition:** People with family members with a history of substance use disorders are more likely to develop them.

- ☐ **Mental health disorders:** Having a diagnosis such as depression, anxiety, and PTSD can increase the risk of substance use disorder.

- ☐ **Childhood trauma:** Traumatic experiences during childhood, such as abuse, neglect, or witnessing violence, can increase the risk of substance use disorder later in life.

- ☐ **Peer pressure:** Being around people who use drugs or alcohol can increase the likelihood of substance use and eventual substance misuse.

- ☐ **Environment:** Factors such as poverty, unemployment, and lack of support can increase the risk of substance use disorder.

- ☐ **Isolation and lack of social support:** Sometimes we use because we're lonely and we don't see any other way to deal with the stress, and that use becomes problematic.
- ☐ **Age of first use:** Individuals who begin using drugs or alcohol at a young age are more likely to develop addiction later in life.

While these risk factors increase an individual's likelihood of developing a substance use disorder, they do not guarantee it. And people without any known risk factors can also develop substance use disorder. These, of course, are not the only risk factors, but they are the most common.

How many risk factors did you have? _____

How do you feel about your risk factors? _____

_____

_____

_____

_____

_____

The Impacts of Substance Use Disorder

Substance use disorder can affect you in many ways. It can impact your physical health, cause emotional stress, damage relationships, create financial strain, and even affect your spirituality and your sense of yourself. These effects can also be compounded by a trauma history.

Impact on Physical and Emotional Health

Substance use can lead to a wide range of physical complications—liver failure, respiratory problems, heart disease, high blood pressure, and skin infections, to name a few. Many of these issues are caused by years of substance misuse, but not always. A person who uses IV drugs, for example, can get infections, hepatitis C, or HIV, caused by reusing or sharing needles.

Substance use can also cause considerable emotional strain. For some of us, it causes or exacerbates mental health issues. For instance, substance use can sometimes worsen or cause anxiety, depression, and even psychosis. It also makes it increasingly difficult to seek help or treatment for these issues (Ouimette, Goodwin, and Brown 2006)

We'll explore the consequences of substance use—and trauma—on your emotional health in more depth in later chapters. For now, take a second to write some initial thoughts and observations about how your substance use has affected your physical and emotional health.

_____

_____

_____

_____

_____

_____

Impact on Family

Family members may feel helpless, sad, or angry watching their loved one struggle with substance use disorder. Sometimes, family members may believe they are helping by providing financial support or covering up for the individual's behavior, but these actions can prolong the problem. Additionally, substance use disorder can lead to legal issues, health problems, and even death, which can profoundly impact family members.

Family members may experience feelings of guilt, shame, anger, and confusion regarding a loved one's use. Stigma can make these family members feel isolated and unwilling to share details of their loved one's substance use, which may prevent them from seeking their own support. Substance use can also lead to strained relationships, as family members may struggle to trust and communicate with the person who is using.

It is hard to look at how our substance use has affected our family. We often feel deep shame, which can cause more using of substance to drown out those uncomfortable feelings. As hard as it may seem, it is important to take an honest look at how your actions have affected your loved ones. How has your substance use impacted your family?

_____

_____

_____

_____

_____

_____

_____

Financial Impact

Substance use disorder is often accompanied by financial difficulties. The costs of obtaining and using substances, including alcohol, can quickly add up. This is especially true if the person develops a tolerance and needs to use more to get the same effect they did at a lower amount.

Misuse of substances can impact one's employment. It can lead to decreased productivity, absenteeism, and tardiness, resulting in job loss or disciplinary action even if one does not engage in substance use while at work. It can cause individuals to make poor decisions and engage in risky behavior, leading to workplace accidents and injuries. Sometimes individuals may resort to illegal activities to obtain the money needed to support their substance use, which can further exacerbate their financial troubles and add legal issues.

Have you ever considered how using substances has impacted your finances? Over time, the cost of any substance takes a toll on your bank account. Take smoking cigarettes, for example. The average price of a pack of cigarettes at the time of writing is $8 in the U.S. Cigarettes are almost double that in some states, but for this example, we will say they cost $8 (World Population Review 2024). The average smoker will consume twenty cigarettes per day, or one pack. If you calculate $8 a day for a thirty-day month, that is a cost of $240 per month. If you calculate for an entire year, that is a cost of $2,880, which does not include the cost to your health. Smokers are more likely to become ill with respiratory illness, so if you add in the healthcare cost, that increases the cost even more.

Take a moment to consider how using substances has affected your financial life:

What are all the types of substances you have used? _____

_____

_____

_____

_____

_____

How often did/do you use those substances? _____

_____

_____

_____

_____

What is or was the average cost of those substances?

How much does that calculate to per year?

How has your substance use impacted your or someone else's financial situation?

Have you faced legal consequences as a result of substance use? If so, what was the cost of that experience?

Last, how else can you spend the money you have used on substance use?

Spiritual Impact

For many people, spirituality or religion are important in their lives. "Spirituality" is a concept that refers to an individual's inner life, beliefs, values, and experiences. It is often associated with feelings of meaning, purpose, and connection to something larger than oneself. "Religion" refers to a set of beliefs, practices, and rituals that are associated with a particular faith or community (Arrey et al. 2016). Religion often has shared beliefs and values passed down through generations and can provide a sense of community and belonging.

There are several ways that spirituality and substance affect each other. Some people may have religious or spiritual trauma. (Remember that trauma is the emotional response to something that is distressing and difficult to cope with.) Other people experience guilt, shame, or self-blame about how they may have behaved, as substance use can cause people to act in ways they normally would not—ways that go against their values and beliefs. You may also have used substances to cope with spiritual distress or fill a perceived spiritual void, which just worsened the substance use disorder. Addressing the spiritual effects substance use has caused in your life is, for many, an important part of the recovery process.

Consider how your substance use has affected your sense of self. Has it affected your behavior—leading you to act in ways that have caused you guilt, shame, or not being enough? Have you used substances to cope with spiritual distress or fill a perceived spiritual void? Keep in mind the goal here is not to worsen these feelings; it's to begin understanding and articulating what you feel so you can work to heal it.

Conclusion

Substance use disorder is a disease that can affect many areas of one's life, and therefore, is a health issue. Over time, substance use disorder can lead to health complications; it can also cause or worsen anxiety, psychosis, depression, and other mood disorders. Similarly, there are physical responses to trauma that include having headaches, stomach pain and digestive issues, difficulty falling asleep or staying asleep, racing heart and sweating, and being easily startled. (National Institute of Mental Health 2024)

Before recovery, there can also be social and financial difficulties from job loss, financial strain, and strained relationships. Legal troubles can arise from drug-related crimes, such as possession or driving under the influence. Substance use disorders can also be influenced by trauma or the result of trauma.

There are over 20 million adults in the U.S. who identify as being in recovery from a mental health disorder, including the impacts of trauma and or a substance use disorder. (Substance Abuse and Mental Health Services Administration 2023) This workbook is about meeting your unique needs as someone who has experienced trauma and problematic substance use, so we'll explore this further in the next chapter and beyond. I am so glad that you are one of the people who have chosen recovery for yourself.

Chapter 2

What Is Trauma?

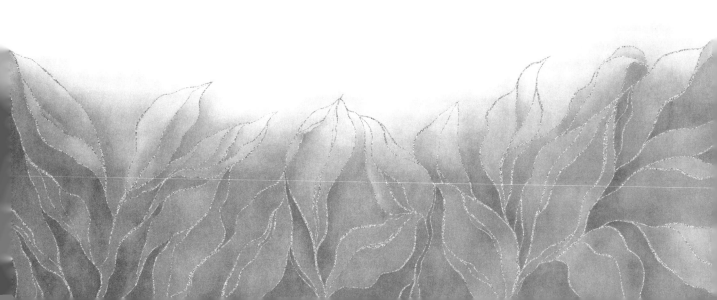

In this chapter, we'll explore the concept of trauma—what it is, how it can affect the brain and behavior, the effects it may have had on your life, and some basic strategies for dealing with those effects when they manifest—as preparation for the work of healing and recovery you'll do working with this book.

Defining Trauma

When we think of someone experiencing trauma, we might think of a combat veteran and everything they have experienced, or of someone who has been through a brutally intense physical or emotional experience. There may also be a belief that unless you have a diagnosis of PTSD, your trauma is "not that bad" or "is not really considered trauma." The reality is that there are many experiences that can cause trauma, and not all trauma comes with a diagnosis.

PTSD, as a diagnosis, is often given to people who have had exposure to death—threatened death, actual or threatened serious injury, or actual or threatened sexual violence. The exposure may be a direct experience of these things, but it does not have to be. You might witness an event and be just as traumatized as someone who experienced it, in a phenomenon called secondary or vicarious trauma.

Learning about the traumatic events of a family member or close friend can also constitute a secondary trauma, as can repeated exposure to details of traumatic events (which is often the case in certain lines of work, such as social workers and first responders).

Ultimately, there are three main types of trauma (Feriante and Sharma 2023):

- Acute trauma resulting from a single incident

- Chronic trauma, which is repeated and prolonged—an example would be domestic violence or abuse

- Complex trauma, which is exposure to varied and multiple traumatic events, often of an invasive, interpersonal nature

Trauma has many effects. Some of the symptoms that people with PTSD experience are intrusive memories, distressing dreams about the event, flashbacks, psychological distress at exposure to cues that symbolize or resemble an aspect of the trauma, avoidance, inability to remember aspects of the trauma, self-blame, negative emotional state, diminished interest in significant activities, feelings of detachment, and inability to experience positive emotions. People with a diagnosis of PTSD can also experience one or more of the following: irritable behavior and angry outbursts, reckless or self-destructive behavior, hypervigilance, exaggerated startle response, problems with concentration, sleep disturbance (American Psychiatric Association 2013).

Ultimately, though, this workbook is for people who have a substance use disorder *and* have experienced trauma—exposure to an incident or a series of emotionally disturbing or life-threatening events that has lasting adverse effects on a person's functioning and well-being. You may or may not have a diagnosis of PTSD, but that will not matter as you work your way through the workbook. Living through a house fire or a car accident can be traumatic. People involved in serious car accidents are at an increase for experiencing PTSD (Beck and Coffey 2007). Anytime someone believes there is a threat of death, or injury, there is risk of developing PTSD. It is not about the severity of the situation but how it affects you.

The Brain and Trauma

When someone experiences trauma, it can have both short-term and long-term effects on the brain. When someone is experiencing a traumatic event, their brain can become overwhelmed, making it difficult to recall what happened later. Trauma can also cause changes that have long-term effects in certain brain structures, specifically the amygdala, hippocampus, and prefrontal cortex.

The amygdala helps regulate emotions, including fear, anxiety, and aggression. It also plays a role in processing and remembering emotional events. Trauma can cause the amygdala to become hyperactive, leading to increased fear and anxiety even in nonthreatening situations.

The hippocampus is the part of the brain that deals with learning and storing memories. It is also involved in the regulation of emotions. Changes in the hippocampus can cause memory loss and other cognitive impairments. Trauma can cause the hippocampus to shrink in size. This can lead to difficulties with memory and even increase the risk of developing PTSD.

The prefrontal cortex is the part of the brain that deals with decision making, personality expression, and social behavior. Trauma can impair its function, leading to difficulties with impulse control and emotional regulation and even greater risk-taking behavior.

One of the first steps in healing from your trauma is understanding what it is and what may have caused it. Below is a list of traumatic experiences. Put a check mark next to the ones that you have experienced.

Experiences that may be traumatic include:

- ☐ Physical, sexual, and emotional abuse
- ☐ Seeing a loved one experience abuse
- ☐ Witnessing or experiencing intimate partner violence
- ☐ Being in or witnessing combat
- ☐ Childhood neglect
- ☐ Living with a family member with mental health or substance use disorders
- ☐ Sudden, unexplained separation from a loved one
- ☐ Poverty
- ☐ Racism, discrimination, homophobia, and oppression
- ☐ Being bullied
- ☐ Violence in the community, war, or terrorism
- ☐ Natural disasters, such as hurricanes, earthquakes, and floods
- ☐ Loss of a home
- ☐ Surviving a family member dying by their own hand
- ☐ Witnessing someone being killed
- ☐ Car crashes or other accidents

- ☐ Community and school violence
- ☐ Exposure to traumatic events at work
- ☐ Chronic stress
- ☐ Other _____

Were you aware of the number of traumatic events that you have experienced? _____

What were those experiences like for you? _____

_____

_____

_____

Unpacking and looking at your trauma can be difficult. Take a few moments and write and reflect on what you are feeling.

_____

_____

_____

_____

_____

_____

_____

• *Mary's Story*

Mary is a twenty-five-year-old single female who lives in a small apartment building in the city. She loves the location of her apartment as it is close to public transportation, grocery stores, and the gym. She works from home as an editor and loves her job. She has friends and likes going out to dinner and the theater with them.

One afternoon as Mary returns from brunch with her girlfriends, she notices fire trucks on her street. As she gets closer, she sees that the firefighters are just getting done putting out a fire that has gutted the entire building.

Mary is in shock, as everything except what she has on her was lost in the fire. She calls her mother, who lives three hours away, and tells her what has happened. Since Mary does not have a car, her mother drives the three hours to come pick her up.

Mary decides to wait at a nearby bar for her mother to arrive and order a drink. She is alone at the bar; she can think only of everything she has lost. During the three-hour wait, Mary drinks many more drinks than she intended. By the time her mother arrives, Mary is intoxicated. When Mary gets in her mother's car, she starts crying. Her mother drives her back to her home. Mary does not want anything to eat and goes to bed.

It may not seem realistic that someone could experience trauma resulting from property loss, but this is something that can be very traumatizing for people. Mary's choice to go to a bar to wait for her mom and have drinks may not have been the best choice she could have made. For instance, she had friends in the city; she could have waited for her mom with one of them and gotten some support too.

As we move through this chapter, we will return to Mary and her story to discover how the experience of trauma can intersect with and sometimes worsen substance use issues.

Aftereffects of Trauma

Experiencing trauma can cause many symptoms or aftereffects. These symptoms can vary from person to person and can impact a wide range of areas in your life. Below is a list of some common aftereffects. Put a check mark next to the ones that you have experienced:

- ☐ Anxiety
- ☐ Depression
- ☐ Avoidance
- ☐ Anger
- ☐ Irritability
- ☐ Mood swings
- ☐ Feeling overwhelmed
- ☐ Arousal and reactivity (this can present as a low startle response)
- ☐ Numbness, a sense of detachment or disconnection from others
- ☐ Unpredictable emotions
- ☐ Difficulty concentrating
- ☐ Loss of interest in activities
- ☐ Sleep disturbances
- ☐ Nightmares, flashbacks
- ☐ Physical symptoms such as headaches, nausea, and fatigue, and changes in appetite
- ☐ Other _____

Looking at the aftereffects you experience, which ones cause you the most discomfort?

_____

_____

_____

Mary's Story, Continued

The next morning, Mary is numb. She has no idea what to do. Her mother tries to help her document her losses, obtain a fire report, and call her insurance company; among other things, she suggests that Mary call work and let them know what happened. Mary calls her job and tells them about the fire and that the company laptop was destroyed. Her supervisor tells her that she will send another out to her mother's house, but it will take about a week to arrive. She suggests that Mary take vacation time while waiting for the new laptop.

On the call, Mary agrees; she doesn't feel she has much choice. But she becomes very angry when telling her mother about the call: "I just lost everything, and she is making me take my vacation time. I was going to use my vacation time this winter to go skiing with my friends." The more Mary's mom attempts to comfort her, the angrier she becomes. Mary goes to her childhood bedroom and begins to cry.

In the coming days and weeks, Mary finds herself having difficulty concentrating and often sits at her computer for long stretches of time just staring at the screen. What once came so easy is now very difficult, and she no longer enjoys her work.

Mary starts having difficulty falling asleep, so she starts making herself a drink at night to help her sleep. She often wakes in the middle of the night after having dreams about the fire and cannot fall back asleep. She starts drinking to get herself back to sleep. Quickly her nightly drinks turn into a nightly bottle of wine, followed by more drinks in the night if she wakes.

Mary, who had always been very easygoing, finds herself often snapping at her mother. After doing so, she feels bad and cries, saying, "I am so mean, I do not know what is wrong with me."

As you can likely tell, Mary is experiencing several aftereffects in the days and weeks after the apartment fire. She no longer enjoys what she once did and lacks the concentration she once had. She finds she's getting frustrated with herself and her mother, with whom she had to move back in. And she doesn't understand why she's feeling and acting the way she is.

The aftereffects of trauma can be difficult to deal with. Learning skills on how to deal with these symptoms is an important step in healing. People who have had one or more traumatic events may have times when they feel like they are not emotionally stable, well-balanced, or able to remain calm and rational in the face of stress or adversity. This feeling is often referred to as being "ungrounded" or "needing to become grounded." When you feel ungrounded, you may also feel scattered, anxious, or overwhelmed, and struggle to stay focused or make rational decisions.

Being grounded, by contrast, is a feeling of being connected to reality and having a clear and realistic sense of one's own strengths and limitations. When you are grounded, you are more centered, focused, and able to make sound decisions.

Grounding

There are several ways that you can become grounded when you sense you've become ungrounded. Of course, when you get out of balance, your brain has a difficult time functioning optimally and recall may not be easy. The exercise that follows, the 5-4-3-2-1 exercise, is an especially useful technique because it is easy to remember.

Name five things you can see.

1. _____
2. _____
3. _____
4. _____
5. _____

Name four things you can touch right now.

1. _____
2. _____
3. _____
4. _____

Name three things you hear right now.

1. _____
2. _____
3. _____

Name two things you can smell right now.

1. _____
2. _____

Name one thing you can taste.

1. _____

As you reflect on the 5-4-3-2-1 exercise, describe how you think this tool could be helpful to you in times of stress.

_____
_____
_____
_____
_____

    Counting shapes is another grounding skill that can be easily remembered anywhere. This is my personal favorite because you have to remember only one thing: rectangles. Take a look around the space you are currently in and see how many rectangles you can count. Much like the previous exercise, refocusing your attention on something else distracts your brain from the thoughts and emotions that are causing you to feel ungrounded. If you are in a nature setting such as a park, rectangles may be difficult to find. I encourage you to count instead the number of green things, or rocks, or flowers that you see.

Take a look around the space you are currently in and see how many rectangles you can count. They are everywhere!

How many did you find? _____

Childhood Experiences

The adverse relationships and experiences we have in childhood can have a lasting effect on our health and well-being. Understanding the number of these experiences can give you a fuller picture of how they may impact your life now. Take your time in completing the questions about your adverse childhood experiences (ACEs) below (Jackson Nakazawa 2024). Put a check mark next to any item you experienced before your eighteenth birthday:

- ☐ Physical neglect—not having enough to eat, having to wear dirty clothes, or having no one to protect or take care of you
- ☐ Growing up in poverty or with excessive financial worries
- ☐ Facing medical trauma, either your own or a family member's
- ☐ Loss of a parent, caregiver, family member, or close friend through divorce, abandonment, death, or some other reason
- ☐ Separation from a parent or caregiver for weeks or months, including adoption or foster care
- ☐ Parental depression, mental illness, or attempted suicide
- ☐ Living with someone who had a problem with drinking or using drugs, including

- ☐ prescription drugs

- ☐ Witnessing a parent being abused—hitting, punching, beating, or threatening to harm each other

- ☐ Having an incarcerated family member

- ☐ Having a parent or adult swear at you, insult you, or put you down

- ☐ Facing racism or discrimination

- ☐ Having a parent or adult in your home ever hit, beat, kick, or physically hurt you

- ☐ Chronic bullying from siblings or peers

- ☐ Growing up in a violent neighborhood

- ☐ Feeling that no one in your family loved you or thought you were special or that your family didn't support each other

- ☐ Unwanted sexual contact

- ☐ Facing an environmental crisis or disaster such as an earthquake, wildfire, flood, tornado, hurricane, or pandemic

How many items did you check off? _____

The more boxes you checked, the higher your risk of physical and psychological conditions or experiences later in life—conditions such as substance use disorder, depression, heart disease, or chronic obstructive pulmonary disease (COPD), or experiences such as the early initiation of sexual activity, intimate partner violence, sexually transmitted diseases or STIs, or suicide attempts. It is important to note that a high score does not guarantee you will have these experiences; it's simply an index of potential increased risk (U.S. Centers for Disease Control and Prevention 2024).

Questionnaires like these are also a good way to recognize what trauma can do to the body and mind if it is overlooked. Completing a questionnaire like this and contemplating the effects of ACEs may have been an intense experience. The key to keep in mind is that by addressing the aftereffects of trauma, you can lower your risk factors for the future.

Protective Factors

Protective factors are characteristics that lower the likelihood of adverse outcomes or reduce the impact of risk factors (CDC 2024). They can be considered positive countermeasures. Even if you have many risk factors, you may also have experienced some protective factors that improve your resilience to adverse experiences:

- ☐ Caregivers created safe, positive relationships with you.
- ☐ Another adult cared for you and was someone you felt safe with.
- ☐ Caregivers met your basic needs of food, shelter, education, and health services.
- ☐ Families had strong social support networks and stable, positive relationships with the people around them.
- ☐ Your family was present and interested in you as child.
- ☐ Your household had rules and engaged in monitoring you.
- ☐ You had safe, stable housing growing up.
- ☐ You lived in a community where families have access to nurturing and safe childcare.
- ☐ You got medical care and mental health services.

How many checkmarks did you have? _____

This is your protective factor score. A score of 3 is "average resilience," while a score of 5 or more marks "high resilience."

Keep in mind that no matter your score, the fact that you are working on this workbook shows that you want to recover from the difficulties you have experienced. Whether this comes easily, or you have to work at it, does not matter. What matters is that you are on a journey of recovery.

Conclusion

Whether you have experienced a traumatic event or several traumatic events, these can affect your mental health and well-being. Ignored trauma can lead to anxiety, depression, flashbacks, nightmares, and substance use. Recovering from your trauma is important because it allows you to learn coping skills to manage the aftereffects of trauma—ones that don't involve problematic substance use—and work toward healing.

By acknowledging your trauma and looking at the effects it has had on your life, you can gain a sense of control and empowerment over your life. You may also be able to reduce the impact that your trauma may have on your physical health in the years to come.

Recovery from trauma is not an event, but rather a journey. I am very grateful that you have decided to either start or continue that journey for yourself. In the next chapter, we'll continue that journey by exploring how trauma and substance use are interrelated.

Chapter 3

The Connection Between Trauma and Substance Use Disorder

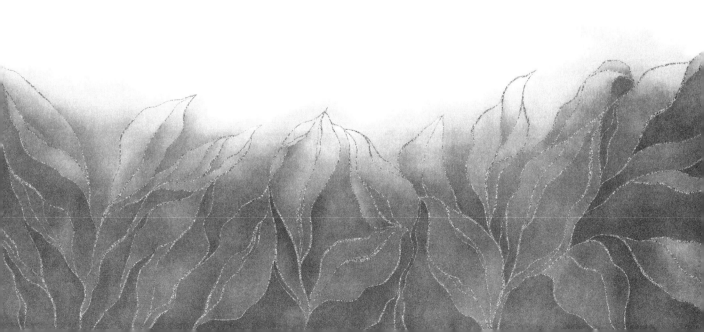

As I indicated in the introduction, experiencing trauma is a risk factor for substance misuse and substance misuse puts one at risk for experiencing traumatic events. These two are closely linked. Some people start misusing substances after experiencing a traumatic event. Others may start with a habit of substance use that eventually exposes them to trauma. People with a substance use disorder may find themselves in a cycle in which exposure to traumatic events produces increased alcohol and drug use, which produces new exposure to more traumatic events, which influences further substance use, and the cycle goes on and on.

An example of this might be the person whose inhibitions become lowered when they use substances, and they then engage in risky behavior they would not otherwise engage in, putting themselves at risk of experiencing a traumatic event. They may then start to use more substances to numb those feelings or "medicate" their trauma.

In this chapter, we'll begin to explore the effects that combined substance use and trauma may have had on your life. We'll consider different approaches to recovery from substance use, namely abstinence and harm reduction, to determine which is the better choice for you. We will also look at the effects of trauma you may still be dealing with today and how you might be able to respond to those effects differently, with more adaptive coping mechanisms. Finally, we'll also look at your stress levels, which can affect your well-being and your recovery from substance use and trauma, to see if you might be able to reduce those.

Abstinence or Harm Reduction?

Not everyone who misuses substances wants to stop using substances. Some people may find that they want to stop using one type of substance. Perhaps they want to continue to use a substance, but they want to limit the negative impact that use can have on their lives. This is a form of what's known as harm reduction—the practice of reducing the negative consequences that might be associated with substance use rather than eliminating use altogether.

• Sadie's Story

Drinking had been a part of Sadie's life since her mid-twenties. When she was in her thirties, she started using cocaine. She found that it helped her stay awake, so she was able to get more things done. Her occasional use of cocaine quickly turned to daily use. Shortly after that, she started going to the bar every night after work. There, she would often drink more alcohol than she intended. The cocaine also allowed her to drink more since she wouldn't get tired. Driving home one night after an evening of drinking and using cocaine, she hit a lamp post. She was not seriously hurt, but she did get arrested for driving under the influence.

The next morning, waking up in jail, Sadie continued to have flashbacks to the night before. A friend had died in a drunk driving accident a few years before, and it had been very hard on Sadie at the time. Now, she kept having thoughts of what would have happened if she had killed someone and remembering the pain of losing her friend. She wasn't able to sleep for several days after the accident and became anxious. Ultimately, she missed several days of work because she was unable to focus due to lack of sleep. She then had the added stress of the financial burden of replacing her car and paying legal fees.

In the wake of the incident, Sadie realized that her misuse of substances had brought on all these issues. And she realized she truly did not want to be responsible for bringing herself or someone else to grievous harm. Realistically, she also did not see herself stopping entirely either. Sadie decided she would stop using all substances except alcohol. She still went to the bar, but only a few times a week. She also held herself to a commitment: She would go home and drop off her car, then walk to the bar to drink, so she would not drink and drive.

Sadie's substance misuse caused a traumatic event that rippled into many other areas of her life and caused unpleasant consequences. The accident also resurfaced the trauma of losing her friend years earlier. For her and others' health and safety, Sadie needed to decide how she would change her substance use.

Abstinence-only recovery is a path for some people, but not everyone wants to discontinue using all substances. Using harm reduction as a path to recovery is also valid. For some people, harm reduction might look like stopping using one substance but continuing using another. For example, someone may stop using cocaine, but find they can drink without it being problematic for them. Another person might continue using a substance, but either reduce their frequency of use or set up structures to reduce potential harm. For example, I drink caffeine to excess. I know this creates several issues, and yet, I still want to drink it. One thing I started to do was to not drink any caffeinated beverages past 6 p.m. Doing this one thing allows me to sleep better at night, which helps me the next day in a number of ways. This, too, is a form of harm reduction.

In Sadie's example above, she did both. She did not want to have all the negative effects of her substance use—but she did not want to give it up entirely either. So, she took steps to lessen the impact of her substance use in three different ways. She no longer mixed her drinking with cocaine use, she decreased the number of nights she would go out drinking, and she put measures into place to prevent her from driving home from the bar after drinking. By taking these steps, she reduced the harm of both her substance use and her trauma.

No matter what your recovery path is, think about some action steps you can take to lessen the negative effects of things you may be doing at this time in your life.

Big T and Little T Trauma

As we think about trauma, it can be placed into two categories: big T and little t trauma. Big T trauma are those events that are perceived to be life threatening. These events have a sudden and overwhelming impact. Some examples of big T traumas are sexual abuse or assault, witnessing a murder, natural disaster, or acts of terrorism. Little t trauma refers to the repetition or accumulation of less obvious distressing experiences. Some examples of little t trauma include ongoing emotional abuse, neglect, bullying, chronic illness, divorce, constant criticism, and chronic stress (Castillo 2022).

The distinction between the big T and little t trauma is not always clear, and I do not want to diminish your or anyone's experience with trauma in establishing it.

It is important to understand little t trauma and how to cope with it, because it can be easy to ignore. And when it is ignored, it can lead to unhealthy coping mechanisms, including substance misuse.

Maladaptive Coping Mechanisms

People who have experienced trauma and have not worked through it are at risk of developing maladaptive coping mechanisms. This is sometimes referred to as switching one addiction for another. These behaviors may seem helpful and help you avoid discomfort, but in the long run, can cause you more harm.

- *Jane's Story*

    Jane had several adverse childhood experiences and began using substances very early. She then entered recovery in her twenties. Jane never acknowledged that what she had been through, including a sexual assault, was traumatizing. Once she stopped using substances, she started emotionally eating. She felt bad about the effects on both her body and her state of mind, but she continued to overeat to soothe herself. She also found herself going to the casino to play slot machines as another way to prevent herself from feeling her feelings. As she lost more and more of her savings, she became more anxious, which caused her to want to avoid those negative feelings more than ever.

She started working a second job to compensate for her gambling losses. Being overcommitted and busy all the time helped for a short time, but soon she found that it did not work to elevate her feelings.

Look at the maladaptive coping mechanisms below and check the ones that have applied to you, currently or in the past:

- ☐ Substance and alcohol misuse
- ☐ Disordered eating, including bulimia and anorexia
- ☐ Gambling
- ☐ Internet addiction or gaming
- ☐ Overexercising
- ☐ Sex addiction
- ☐ Excessive sleeping
- ☐ Shopping or overspending
- ☐ Self-harm
- ☐ Avoidance
- ☐ Isolation
- ☐ Impulsive or risky behaviors
- ☐ Excessive screen time
- ☐ Staying overly busy
- ☐ Other _____

Look at what you have checked. What are the unhealthy coping mechanisms you want to remove?

_____

_____

_____

_____

What do you envision your life to be like once you no longer rely on unhealthy coping mechanisms?

_____

_____

_____

_____

_____

_____

_____

Activators

People who have experienced trauma and substance use disorders are sometimes triggered—faced with stimuli that bring them back to memories of their traumatic experiences. For some people, the term "triggered" is itself "triggering." The word "activated" is sometimes used to replace the word "trigger" for this reason. I will use the word "activators" as we move forward.

Activators can be anything that causes a person to remember their trauma or their experience with substances. Activators can be sensory, emotional, or environmental cues that bring back memories, and can include things like sights, sounds, smells, tastes, or physical sensations. Activators can be challenging, as they can cause intense feelings. These feelings can be that of fear, anxiety, distress, or, on the flip side, glorifying "the good old days" of substance use. It is important for individuals to be aware of their activators, and to develop coping strategies and self-care practices to help manage their reactions. It is in taking these steps that people can avoid a recurrence of the symptoms of their substance use and trauma.

There are several types of activators people can experience, including environmental, emotional, behavioral, and psychological (Experience Recovery 2022). Let's take a closer look at each type. Below are a few examples of activators, organized by category. Circle the activators that you have experienced. You can also fill in any activators you know of that may be missing from these lists.

Environmental activators (people, places, things):

- Going to places that remind you of your substance use or trauma
- Spending time with people who actively use drugs or alcohol
- Seeing substance- or trauma-related content on social media, movies, or TV shows
- Loud or abrupt noises

- Certain smells
- Bright lights or darkness
- Other _____

Emotional activators (stress, anxiety, depression):

- Loneliness
- Conflicts with family, friends, and romantic partners
- Feelings of vulnerability or rejection
- Emotional occasions, such as vacations, anniversaries, celebrations, and holidays
- Experiencing financial problems or stress at work
- Anger
- Other _____

Behavioral triggers (routine, habits):

- Getting paid or coming into a lot of money
- Staying up all night
- Going on a trip
- Creating unrealistic expectations for yourself
- Becoming overly hungry or not eating
- Unpredictability or sudden change
- Other _____

Psychological activators (negative thoughts, beliefs):

- Feeling a need to escape from reality
- Thoughts of *I'm not good enough, I am a loser*, and so forth
- Judging yourself harshly for mistakes
- Self-blame for outcomes
- Negative thinking about the past
- Other _____

What matters about activators is not what they activate, but how you reprogram your emotions and reactions to those cues. Some time ago, I used to visit a particular building several times a week as part of my work. One day, an event occurred in the entry to the building, and I was called upon to help the people who lived in the building cope with the event. When I arrived, there were a lot of things I witnessed. Because I have a history of experiencing trauma myself, the visual cues I saw activated me and reminded me of a particular trauma from my youth. The activation was not limited to that day. For weeks afterward, every time I entered the building—which was one I had no choice but to enter—I would remember not only the event that occurred at that building but also the event I had witnessed as a child.

I started to have problems sleeping and eating, and issues with concentration. When I started to think about returning to substance use, I knew I had to do something. It was not an option to stop going to the location, so I had to develop a way to neutralize the space so it would no longer cause me to experience intense feelings of anxiety and fear. What worked for me was not to decrease the number of times I went to the building, but to increase it and to behave differently as I entered the building.

Instead of walking in and looking at the entry, I would look beyond that to the person who checked people in. I would look at her face, and smile as I went in the door. I would greet her and ask her about her day, about the weather, about her kids, about anything. Once I did that, I stopped thinking about what I had seen and instead just focused on that woman. It worked! After only a few visits to the building, I stopped having the fear and anxiety when I went to the building; I slept better; I ate better; and most importantly, I stopped thinking about using substances.

You can apply the same strategy to your activators. Once you are clear on what your activators are, you can start to develop a plan to neutralize those cues. Look again at your activators and pick out up to five that are the most problematic for you. Then, write out what you could do to help yourself with them. For instance, you could choose something specific to focus on, like I did—especially if the activator is something you can't avoid. Or you could come up with an adaptive activity that will help you reregulate yourself when you encounter an activator, whether the dysregulation is connected to trauma triggers or to substance use. If you get stuck doing this exercise, here are some suggestions that other people have found helpful to deal with some of their activators. They may help you with this activity:

- Exercise
- Meditation
- Reading
- Journaling
- Spending time with friends and family who understand your recovery journey
- Taking a nap
- Listening to relaxing music
- Playing with your kids and or pet
- Praying
- Coloring
- Yoga
- Eating a nourishing meal
- Distracting yourself, such as counting shapes
- Relaxation techniques and mindfulness

Activators	What can I do to help myself with this?
1.	
2.	
3.	
4.	
5.	

Keeping an activator diary is a good way to identify, anticipate, and reframe activators in your daily life. When you record details about the activating event (what, who, when, and where), you can find patterns in behavior. By thinking about how you'd like to behave differently, you can practice more effective coping skills when you encounter those activators again, thereby reducing the power of those events. (Experience Recovery 2022).

Below is an example of an activator diary you can use. You can download additional copies of this worksheet, if you find it helpful, at http://www.newharbinger.com/54803. Alternatively, you can use some other format—if you prefer, in a personal journal.

Day	What happened?	What did I do?	What do I want to do differently in the future?

Stressors and Trauma

Everyone experiences stress; each day, our lives are full of things and situations that cause us anxiety or frustration. Most of the time, we can adapt to these situations and be flexible. However, when stress goes on for a long time or is particularly intense, we may feel overwhelmed and unable to cope. These may then develop into little t trauma.

As you progress on your healing journey, it is important to understand the types of stress and how they affect you.

Some of the most common types of stress include:

- **Positive stress:** While everyone experiences stress differently, a little stress is a normal part of life. Holidays, the birth of a child, parties, meeting new people, or getting a new car are all examples of positive stress.

- **Short-term stress:** This is stress that lasts for a few moments or hours. Traffic, arguments with a family member, problems at work or school, and having a limited amount of time to complete tasks are all examples of short-term stress.

- **Tolerable stress:** Tolerable stress turns the body's alert system up higher and for a short time. Examples of this might be divorce, the loss of a family member, or a serious illness.

- **Toxic stress:** The term toxic stress refers to our response to ongoing serious stress. We may feel toxic stress when we face intense, frequent, or prolonged challenges. These can include abuse, domestic violence, neglect, or substance use in the home.

Not only does stress put us at risk for a return to use or a resurfacing of our trauma symptoms, it also impacts our health. Stress can release chemicals that over time can damage our bodies, causing mental and physical complications such as muscle pain, high blood pressure, weakened immune system, digestive problems, headaches, heart disease, anxiety, and depression (WI Department of Health 2024).

What type of things cause you stress? How much you are bothered by them? Can you see how stress can affect your wellness and healing?

Write down the top three things that are causing you stress right now and rate each one from 1 to 10, 1 being minimally stressful and 10 being extremely stressful.

1. _____

   Rating: 1   2   3   4   5   6   7   8   9   10

2. _____

   Rating: 1   2   3   4   5   6   7   8   9   10

3. _____

   Rating: 1   2   3   4   5   6   7   8   9   10

Now, think about what you can do in the next thirty days that can eliminate or reduce those stressors. Not all stressors can be eliminated; morning traffic for instance, is not going to go away just because you need to reduce the stress of commuting to the office. But listening to calming music as you drive, or leaving earlier than usual to avoid the worst of the rush may help reduce the stress you feel about that morning drive, reducing the risk that you'll default to maladaptive coping mechanisms.

_____

_____

_____

_____

_____

_____

_____

At the end of the thirty-day period, come back to this workbook and write about what happened. Were you successful in using the strategies you came up with? Did they help to reduce your stress?

_____

_____

_____

_____

_____

_____

_____

_____

Conclusion

Experiencing trauma and problematic substance use are intertwined. When I complete assessments on clients who are receiving treatment for their substance use disorder, I ask if they have ever experienced abuse (physical, emotional, or sexual) or any other traumatic events. Almost without exception, every single person says yes.

For some people, their "core issue" may be their trauma; for others, it may be their substance use. Whether you experienced trauma that then led to a substance use disorder, or your substance use created situations that caused trauma, what is important to remember is that you need to work on healing from both at the same time. Ignoring either one of them can cause you to have a return of symptoms that can lead to more unhealthy coping strategies or behaviors.

Chapter 4

Embarking on the Road to Recovery

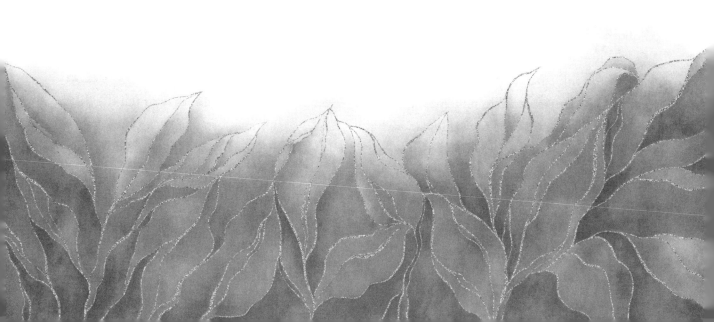

The term "recovery" is often associated with people who are discontinuing their substance use. According to The Substance Abuse and Mental Health Services Administration, recovery is "a process of change that helps people improve their health and wellness, live self-directed lives, and reach their full potential" (SAMHSA 2012).

Notice that SAMHSA's definition does not use the word "substance," nor does it say that someone must have an abstinence-based recovery. As you move forward in this workbook, let us agree that recovery is not limited to one situation or event. When I talk of "recovery," I am referring to not just your substance misuse, or your trauma. I am also referring to a sequence of life changes meant to help you improve your well-being, live life with true agency, and achieve whatever it is you hope to achieve.

When I think about this definition, it is clear to me that this is an inclusive definition that can fit everyone for everything. Whether you are a person who is practicing abstinence-based recovery, wants to reduce your substance use, or is working on healing from trauma, this definition fits you. Remember, there is no "wrong way" to recovery. Everyone wants to reach their full potential, but what that means to me differs from what it does to you.

Your recovery is unique to you and does not have to look the same as everyone else's. The word "recover" means "to get back to." I want you to think of your recovery as more than getting back to where you started. I want you instead to think about working toward the best version of yourself. In this chapter, we'll begin that work by taking stock of where we are and considering the changes we can begin making, particularly in the domain of self-care, to start our path to recovery.

Taking Stock

Taking full stock of your situation is helpful in learning what you're doing that is working and what might need to be removed from your life. Sometimes it is not easy to tell the difference between what is working and what isn't. And sometimes, especially early in recovery, we cannot recognize that what we are doing is not working for us. The reason for our problematic substance use may not be clear to us either.

In the following exercise, you will be invited to think about the times and reasons you have used substances. Take your time filling out the answers. Really reflect on how you have reacted in the past and be as honest as you can. Remember this is about getting a clear idea of how your emotions have led you to ways of coping that you may want to let go of.

Think back to a time when you used drugs or alcohol to cope with difficult emotions, such as stress, anxiety, depression, or trauma. Write about the situation below. What happened? What was it you were trying to avoid? What was the result of your substance use in that moment, in the short term and in the long term?

_____

_____

_____

_____

_____

_____

_____

_____

How often do you or have you used substances to manage your emotions?

_____

_____

_____

Have you ever experienced your feelings intensifying when you use substances? If so, did you feel you were not in control of your feelings or emotions?

Have you ever found it difficult to manage your emotions without relying on substances? What is or was that like for you?

Gambling, eating, sex, excessive exercising or dieting, shopping, and gaming are all examples of behaviors that can become addictive. What other behaviors do you find yourself engaging in to avoid dealing with emotions or feelings?

Do you have healthy coping skills to manage difficult emotions—behaviors that help you deal with difficult emotions and don't have adverse consequences? What are they and how do they help?

_____

_____

_____

_____

_____

If you don't have healthy coping skills, how important do you think it is to develop those skills to avoid substances to manage emotions?

_____

Learning how to deal with your emotions is important in your recovery. In the last chapter, we discussed how trauma and substance misuse are interrelated. The recovery for these two are also interrelated. And it begins with proper self-care.

Self-Care

Taking care of ourselves sounds simple, yet many of us did not take care of ourselves during our substance misuse. In addition to the substances, we may have not eaten well, not exercised enough or regularly, and not gotten significant sleep. Many people who misuse substances also use tobacco. People with a trauma history also use tobacco to distract from their feelings, which can impact health in several ways. Learning to take care of ourselves is something that many of us do for the first time when we enter recovery.

Sleep

Lack of sleep is a common problem and can significantly impact our health. Besides simply feeling tired, not having enough energy to get through the day makes even the simplest tasks seem impossible. Lack of concentration will hinder your speed and accuracy in getting things done and increase your risks of accidents or injury. Other effects of lack of sleep are irritability and mood swings, weakening of the immune system, and an increase in risk-taking behaviors, which can include returning to use (Garbarino et al. 2021; National Heart, Lung, and Blood Institute 2022).

While getting enough sleep can be challenging, prioritizing it is essential. When we're sleep-deprived, our bodies produce more cortisol, which can lead to feelings of anxiety and tension. The reverse is also true: when we get enough sleep, we feel calm, and relaxing is easier. Other benefits of getting enough sleep are improved emotional regulation and mood and decreased depressive symptoms, which lead to overall emotional wellness. We also feel more optimistic when we are well rested.

- *Debbie's Story*

    Debbie experienced many traumatic events in her childhood and teen years. In her early twenties, she misused substances to block out painful memories. Unfortunately, this caused her to make choices that led to more traumatic events, and she became depressed and found it hard to cope, and she was unable to work. After several years, she learned coping skills for her trauma and modified her substance use.

    Soon she was able to go back to work as a truck driver. She was excited to get the opportunity to work again but soon found the inconsistent hours to be problematic. It was hard to establish a regular sleep schedule. Debbie was unable to get the rest her body needed and found that she was tired all the time. She also felt increased anxiety as a result.

    Shortly after that, Debbie started to have intrusive memories of her trauma. And without adequate rest, she was not thinking clearly enough to recall her coping skills in such moments.

    One morning as she was trying to go to sleep in her truck, she started thinking about how using "just a little" would help her sleep. At that point, she realized she was not in a good space and she knew she had to change something; it was not an option for her to use illegal substances and drive a truck, and she did not want to go backwards in her recovery.

She decided to ask for a job working dispatch instead. This would allow her to work a consistent schedule. She also revisited her coping skills and connected with her support system. These steps of self-care helped Debbie be successful in maintaining not only her employment but her recovery as well.

Once Debbie was able to recognize that her lack of self-care regarding her sleep was impacting her recovery, she was able to make some changes to help her adjust.

What is your sleep schedule like? Taking an inventory can be helpful in making the changes you need. Place a check mark next to the steps that you currently take to ensure you are well rested.

- ☐ Stick to a regular sleep schedule by going to bed and waking up at the same time every day.

- ☐ Have a relaxing bedtime routine, such as taking a warm bath, reading a book, or listening to calming music before bed.

- ☐ Avoid caffeine and nicotine, as these things can interfere with sleep and make it harder to fall asleep.

- ☐ Have a comfortable sleep environment by ensuring your bedroom is calm, dark, and quiet.

- ☐ Exercise regularly, as that can help improve sleep quality.

- ☐ Avoid eating heavy meals before bedtime.

How many items did you check? _____

What can you do to increase that number? _____

_____

_____

Other Forms of Self-Care

Of course, there is so much more to self-care than just sleep hygiene. Some other things you can do daily are eat a nutritious and balanced diet, drink enough water throughout the day, move your body regularly through exercise or physical activity, and take breaks. There are also activities you can do to improve your state of mind. These include soothing behaviors like reading something you enjoy, listening to music or a podcast, or spending time outdoors. They also include activities that help you align your life to your values, like setting realistic goals. And they include activities that bolster your support system, like going out to coffee or a meal with a friend, spending regular time with those you love, and other means of staying connected with others with whom you have a supportive and positive relationship.

What things do you do daily that show you practice good self-care?

_____

_____

_____

_____

_____

What are some other self-care activities that you engage in?

_____

_____

_____

_____

What self-care activities would you like to add to your life?

If you find it helpful, you can use the following self-care-activities tracker to begin integrating more and more regular self-care into your life. Each day, write down at least one thing you've done to improve your self-care that day. You might also jot down some brief notes about how each activity made you feel—whether it was helpful or not.

Day	Self-care activity	How it made me feel

Intrusive Thoughts

One challenge many people have is thoughts that they cannot stop; these are called *intrusive thoughts*. An intrusive thought is an unwelcome or involuntary thought, image, or idea that pops up in a person's mind. Intrusive thoughts are normal and are experienced by almost everyone at some point in their lives. Have you ever gotten a song stuck in your head? That is an intrusive thought.

These thoughts, however, can also become problematic and cause distress, anxiety, or discomfort. These thoughts can be disturbing for people in recovery, as the content of these thoughts might be a reminder of their substance use or trauma.

It is important to note that having an intrusive thought does not mean that a person wants to act on it or that they are a bad person. Again, intrusive thoughts are something we all experience. And investing them with too much significance only makes them harder to deal with. It's also true that we can't simply banish them, and trying to make them "go away" can sometimes make them worse, or increase in frequency.

So what can you do when you get a troubling thought stuck in your head? What's more useful than avoiding them is acknowledging that an intrusive thought is present, and guiding your attention elsewhere from there. This is called thought distraction and it's a good way to focus your mind on something else. One such tool is the counting-rectangles exercise that was presented in chapter 2. Another such tool is thought replacement. Thought replacement is different from distraction because you are not just diverting your attention—you are replacing the thoughts you are having with thoughts that are enjoyable. Here is how you use it: When you notice you're having an unwelcome and intrusive thought, first acknowledge that you are having the thought and that it is unwelcome. Next, think of something that you enjoy, and all the steps it takes to complete that task.

Take going fishing for example. Don't just think *I am fishing in my favorite spot*. Instead, think of all the steps you need to take before you even get the line in the water:

1. *I am going to take my red rod and reel and go to my fishing spot.*
2. *I am going to take my reel and click the two pieces together, making sure all the guides are lined up.*
3. *I am going to attach my reel if it is not yet attached.*
4. *I am going to press in the thumb bar to release the line.*
5. *I am going to thread my line through all of the guide holes.*
6. *I am going to attach a hook and worm or lure to the end of my line.*
7. *I am going to place a weight on my line.*
8. *I will put a bobber about eighteen inches from the hook (my personal favorite length based on where I fish).*
9. *I am going to turn the handle on the reel to draw up all the extra line.*
10. *I am going to stand up.*
11. *I will press in the thumb bar and place my rod over my right shoulder.*
12. *I am going to move my right hand forward, releasing the thumb bar at the same time, and watch my hook, line, sinker, and bobber sail in front of me and into the water.*

Who knew there were so many steps to casting a line into the water! Thinking of all the steps helps the mind focus on something else.

I suggest having two thought replacement ideas ready to go before you need them. You can use just about anything as a focus for thought replacement: playing the guitar, painting, knitting, hiking, gardening, working out, playing golf, bowling, riding a horse, even walking the dog. If you do not have any hobbies to draw from yet, don't worry—we will address that later in this workbook. But for now, you can also use something as simple as doing your hair, cooking a meal, setting the table, or washing your car.

What is something you can use in the thought replacement? _____

What are the steps it will take you to do this task?

The next time an intrusive thought arises in your mind, see if practicing the thought replacement exercise or some other form of grounding and attention regulation works to help you tolerate it. Afterward, come back to this workbook and write about the experience. What was it like? What might you want to do differently going forward, if anything?

We all worry from time to time, as it is a natural response to uncertainty. The difference between occasional worry and intrusive thoughts is that, left unchecked, intrusive thoughts can run out of control, and then before you know it, you are living in the future, or in your head, instead of living in the moment.

Living in today does not mean that you do not make plans for the future; however, it does mean that you do not plan the outcome. By not worrying about the outcome of something, you release control over it, and then there is no need to worry. Some examples of things we may worry about and may not have much or any control over are money, employment, relationships, health (yours or others'), our appearance, world events, and politics.

What are some ways that you worry about the what-ifs of life? _____

_____

_____

_____

_____

_____

_____

What are some adaptive ways you might respond instead? Or perhaps, especially when it comes to matters like world events, you might decide what productive action in this sphere might look like for you—as opposed to the unproductive action of obsessive worrying—and commit to that, even as you resolve to spend less time with your worry thoughts.

Conclusion

This chapter is but an introduction to your path to recovery. Hopefully, it will give you some insight into what is possible for you and what it is you want from your recovery.

Keep in mind that the road to recovery is not always easy. It takes work and commitment. However, it's a journey worth taking, as it leads to improved well-being, a better quality of life, and a brighter future.

It's also important to understand that recovery is not a destination but a continuous process. The path to recovery is a personal journey, and what works for one person may not work for another. Hopefully, you will find what works for you and run with it.

Chapter 5

Forgiveness

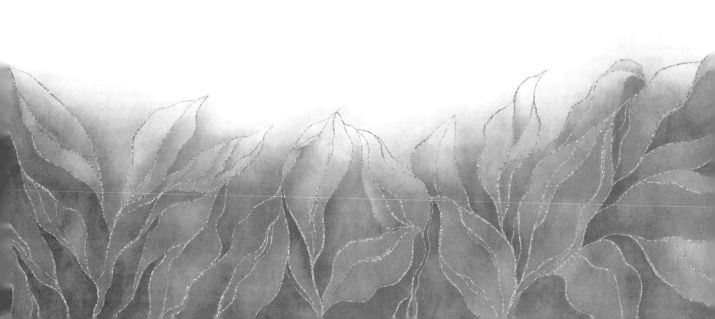

In this chapter, we are going to talk about forgiveness. You may be wondering why we are discussing forgiveness in a workbook about substance use disorder and trauma. The topic of forgiveness can be packed with emotions for people who have had trauma. It's hard to imagine forgiving someone who has caused you pain and trauma. It's helpful to keep in mind that that choice to forgive, or not, is yours.

However, forgiveness can be an important part of recovery. Without it, we can stay stuck in anger, resentment, and pain, all of which are powerful emotions that can lead to a return to use. It may seem impossible to forgive someone, or yourself, for pain (or trauma caused), but you may be surprised how this simple act can change things for you.

At its core, forgiveness is when we intentionally let go of anger and resentment toward someone else who has harmed us. It doesn't mean forgetting, excusing, or condoning the offense, but it does mean you can stop holding so many feelings about it.

Forgiveness can help repair relationships. It can mean that you reconcile with the person who harmed you, but it does not have to. That choice is separate from choosing to forgive them. You have the right to do what feels appropriate and comfortable to you, at any given time.

I want to pay special attention to self-forgiveness. Forgiveness is something we can offer to ourselves no less than others. Self-forgiveness is powerful, and we should not forget about it when we move through this chapter. By forgiving ourselves, we can heal emotionally and move forward. This self-forgiveness will benefit not only us but those around us. As we learn to love and like ourselves, our entire outlook on life improves and our relationships with others are transformed.

The benefits of forgiveness are numerous and can be an important step in reclaiming our lives.

Forgiveness can lead to (Mayo Clinic 2022):

- Healthier relationships
- Improved mental health
- Less anxiety, stress, and hostility
- Fewer symptoms of depression

- Lower blood pressure
- A stronger immune system
- Improved heart health
- Improved self-esteem

When we have not forgiven ourselves or others, not only do we stay stuck in the anger but harboring resentment makes it very difficult to heal. When we cannot heal, we stay stuck in the hurt that was caused, and can end up in a cycle of negative emotions, which can affect our mental and physical health. You may have heard the saying "Resentment is like drinking poison and expecting the other person to die." Learning and practicing forgiveness can be difficult, but it is possible and will certainly help you on your journey of recovery.

How to Forgive

Some people are more forgiving than others, but that does not mean than someone cannot learn to forgive. It is important to remember that if you are stuck in anger and resentment, you are not truly enjoying today. Let's look at one of the first steps to forgiveness.

Acknowledge the Pain

Acknowledging the pain caused is an important step toward forgiveness, as it allows us to face our emotions head-on. When we accept the pain, we validate our feelings and recognize that our feelings are real. Feelings can be overwhelming for a number of reasons. But allowing ourselves to feel them, along with the pain, makes it easier to move on. Feeling all our feelings also allows us to take ownership of our emotions and not project them onto others. By doing this, we can start to process our feelings and work toward healing.

What are some things someone has done to you to cause you pain? How did it make you feel? Are you still feeling that way?

What are some things you have done to cause yourself pain? These might include things you have done to yourself or another person. How did you feel at the time? How do you feel now?

Choose to Forgive

Choosing to forgive can be a difficult decision that requires a great deal of strength and courage. It's important to understand that forgiveness does not mean forgetting what happened. Instead, it's a personal decision to let go of the hurt and anger you've been carrying and release yourself from the emotional burden of holding a grudge.

It's understandable that forgiveness can be challenging, especially when the pain that was caused feels overwhelming. We all have our own unique journey with forgiveness. Your timeline for forgiveness is yours and does not have to look like anyone else's. Forgiveness is not something that can be forced upon us, and it's okay if we're not ready to forgive right away. It's a process, and it may take time to work through our feelings and come to a place of acceptance and peace.

Ultimately, forgiveness is a gift that we give to ourselves. It allows us to move forward and find closure rather than be held back by past hurts and resentments.

Making a commitment to forgive someone is often not a one-and-done event. It may take a long time, and it may be a gradual process.

- *Tony's Story*

Tony had been friends with Alex for years. They served in the military together and later got into recovery together. One day, Alex took some of Tony's tools without asking. Tony mentioned to Alex that he was missing some tools and Alex said, "Oh, I borrowed those." Tony was irritated that Alex would come into his garage without permission and take something without asking, and this was not the first time this had happened.

Tony did not share his feelings, but instead just asked for the tools back. After a week, Alex still had not returned the tools and Tony asked again for the tools to be returned. After a month, Alex still had not given back the tools, and when asked again, he said he had left them at his dad's home, who lived three hours away. Tony felt angry, betrayed, and hurt. He couldn't believe that his friend would be so irresponsible and careless of his feelings.

For weeks, Tony refused to speak to Alex or even entertain the idea of forgiveness. He felt that what Alex had done was unforgivable. The more he thought about it, the angrier he became. One night while thinking about Alex "stealing" his tools and feeling depressed about losing one of his closest friends, he started to think about using again. It was then that Tony began to realize that holding on to his anger and hurt wasn't doing him any good, and might just hurt him. He missed his friend and longed for the bond they shared.

Tony decided to reach out to Alex and arrange a meeting. Alex apologized sincerely and swore that he did not steal the tools, only borrowed them. He had tried to call to set up a time to bring them by after he picked them up from his dad's, but Tony didn't answer the phone. Alex promised to not take things without asking. Tony realized that his friend was truly sorry and that he wanted to make amends.

Tony decided to forgive Alex. He knew that forgiveness didn't mean forgetting the past, but it did mean that he could move forward with love and compassion in his heart. Tony's friend was truly grateful for his understanding and forgiveness, and they both worked hard to rebuild their friendship.

The story is a simple one that reflects what you can gain from forgiveness. Tony chose to forgive Alex not for Alex's benefit, but for his own. Tony allowed his friend Alex to apologize for what he had done, and by doing so, not only did Alex feel better but so did Tony.

One way you can move to a commitment to forgive is to first understand why you want to forgive. What do you have to gain by forgiving the person who has harmed you? What do you have to gain by forgiving yourself? Below is a checklist of some of the reasons you may want to commit to forgive. Check the ones that you think apply for you:

- ☐ Healing
- ☐ Letting go of being the victim
- ☐ Having compassion for self and others
- ☐ Healthier relationships
- ☐ Self-esteem and hope
- ☐ Giving up resentment, revenge, and obsession
- ☐ Serenity

☐ Happiness

☐ Gaining an understanding that everyone is doing the best they can in a given situation or time

What are some other reasons you may have for making the commitment to forgive?

_____

_____

_____

_____

_____

_____

Let Go of Anger and Resentment

We have talked about anger and resentment being the opposite of forgiveness and what lack of forgiveness can lead to—which is why letting go of anger and resentment is so important in moving forward with a more positive and peaceful mindset.

• *Marie's Story*

Doug often was sharp tongued when he drank too much. Doug would often call his family members once he started drinking and say many unkind things to them. Doug usually would not remember what he had said during these calls. After a number of these calls, his sister Marie decided to stop answering the phone. Marie had been in recovery from her own substance use disorder for many years and could not stand to hear her brother being intoxicated and being mean. Doug continued to call his sister, and when she would not pick up, he would leave voice messages. When Doug was not drinking and would call his sister, he could not understand why she did not call him back.

After many months of not talking to her brother and being full of anger, Marie sat down and wrote out her feelings. Once she was done, she saw that her anger in part was fear for her brother and the impact drinking was having on his health. Marie was also able to see that she had not set boundaries with her brother when he had said mean things to her. She was upset with herself about that.

Sometimes, as in the case of Marie, our resentment is not only directed toward someone else but mixed with anger at ourselves. It was by journaling that Marie was able to see that her anger was not only with her brother but herself as well.

One of the best ways to release emotions and get to the core of things is through journaling. Writing down your feelings and thoughts can help you understand why you're feeling what you are. You might find that you're holding on to anger or resentment toward someone who has hurt you, or maybe you're upset with yourself for something you did or didn't do. Whatever the case, writing it down can help you work through those emotions and let them go.

What thoughts and emotions come to mind when you think about a specific situation in which you were harmed?

_____

_____

_____

_____

_____

_____

Talking to a friend or provider can also be incredibly helpful in releasing negative emotions. Sometimes, having someone to talk to makes all the difference. A friend or therapist can provide a listening ear and offer valuable insights and advice. They might help you see things differently and find new ways to cope with your emotions.

In chapter 10, Recovery Planning, we will expand on the concept of who your support people are. For now, who are some people you can talk to who will help you release negative emotions and not intensify them?

_____

_____

_____

_____

_____

Communicate

• *Hanna's Story*

Hanna sent a text to her friend Louise one day and asked her how she was doing and to give her a call. After about an hour, Hanna could see that Louise had read the message, but she had not replied. While Hanna waited for a call or a reply, she became mad that Louise had not called her or even returned her text. As the days passed, Hanna became convinced that Louise was mad at her.

After three days, Hanna finally called Louise and asked her why she had never called or returned the text. Louise apologized and told Hanna that she had been very busy at work, and on top of that, her daughter was sick. Louise acknowledged that she had seen the text and was going to return it later, and then forgot.

Sometimes, but not always, the reasons we are hurt by someone are misunderstandings or miscommunication. When this is the case, communication is helpful in resolving it.

It is not necessary to talk to the person who has harmed you to forgive them. In some situations, it may cause you more harm if you initiate a conversation with them. Weigh the pros and cons before you decide if you want to communicate with them. Each person's situation and circumstances and different, and it is okay to decide not to communicate with a person directly if you don't think it's emotionally or physically safe.

For me, self-forgiveness is one of the most important things I have done, and it became possible with self-communication. I remember the day that the journey of self-forgiveness started. I was taking a coaching class, and the topic was forgiveness. We were given the assignment to write a letter to the person who had harmed us. As I thought about the person who I believed had been the reason for my difficulties, I started my letter. After only one paragraph, my writing shifted, and I was writing the letter to my past self. I wrote down my actions and what they had caused, how those actions harmed not only me but also the people who were close to me. By the time I finished the letter, I was writing that I forgave myself and that I had truly done the best I could at the time. I was crying as I folded my letter. We went out into the yard and burned them in a fire pit. It was one of the most liberating moments of my recovery.

Write a letter to your past self. You can use the space in this workbook, a separate sheet of paper, or a downloadable page to write on at the website for this book, http://www.newharbinger.com/54803.

Once you are done with the letter, you may want to release it as I did, by tearing it up or burning it, or you may want to keep it to look back on and reflect. There is no right or wrong way to let go and move on. Do what feels right to you at this time.

Now, think about if you would like to talk with a person who has harmed you. Take a few moments to think about what you would like to say. Often in an exercise like this, it is best to do a first draft, as many of your feelings are likely to come out. One tip is to identify behaviors that felt harmful and use "I" statements to name what you were feeling, for example, "When you yell at me, I feel scared." Feel free to write what you feel here or print another copy of the lined paper for letter writing at the website, http://www.newharbinger.com/54803.

How to Know If You've Forgiven Someone

Recognizing signs of forgiveness is an important step in the healing journey. It's not always easy to know if you've truly forgiven someone. Below are some indicators that you have forgiven someone (Reinert 2021):

- You no longer hold a grudge or anger toward the person who hurt you. Instead, you may feel a sense of peace or acceptance about the situation.

- You have let go of the negative emotions and moved on from the pain you once felt.

- You no longer obsess over what happened and can focus on other aspects of your life.

Have you let go of the anger you have held about the person or situation that you want to forgive? What are your indicators that you no longer are angry?

_____

_____

_____

_____

If the person is still in your life and you choose to have a relationship with them, you may feel that your relationship with them has improved, or you may have gained a better understanding of them. You may feel more empathetic toward them. This new understanding can lead to a stronger relationship with the person. Remember, it's okay not to have a relationship with someone who has harmed you. That is not a requirement of forgiveness.

Do you have an improved relationship with the person that harmed you? If you are working on self-forgiveness, are you kinder to yourself? How does that look like for you?

_____

_____

_____

_____

_____

_____

At this point in your journey, you may be able to think about the person or the situation without feeling intense emotional pain. You may still feel sadness or regret but are no longer overwhelmed with negative emotions. You can reflect on what happened without seeking revenge or holding on to anger. You have accepted what happened and can move on without the past holding you back.

Has the pain lessened, or maybe is it even gone? What do you feel when you think of the pain that has been or will be released once you have forgiven?

_____

_____

_____

_____

Conclusion

Forgiveness is a powerful tool that can help us to move on from difficult situations. It is not always easy to forgive, but it is possible. By acknowledging the hurt, choosing to forgive, letting go of negative emotions, communicating, and moving forward, we can experience the healing power of forgiveness and have a richer recovery.

Chapter 6

Self-Esteem

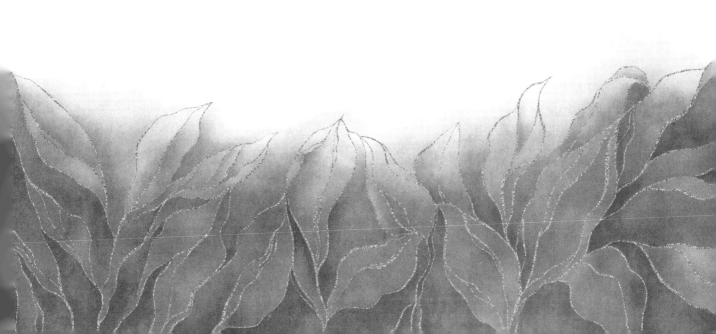

In this chapter, we are going to talk about self-esteem. Self-esteem refers to a person's subjective evaluation of their worth or value: their beliefs about themselves, their abilities, and their attributes. Self-esteem can have an impact on our thoughts, emotions, and behaviors (Schwartz 2020). People with high self-esteem tend to have a positive outlook on life, feel capable of handling challenges, and are more resilient to setbacks. In contrast, people with low self-esteem may struggle with feelings of inadequacy and have negative beliefs about themselves; they may also be more prone to developing a substance use disorder and have fewer skills to deal with the impact of traumatic events.

There is a strong connection between self-esteem and substance use disorder. People with low self-esteem often experience anxiety and depression. As a result, they are more likely to turn to substances as a way of coping with negative emotions, feelings of inadequacy, and insecurities. Substance use, and the context in which it often occurs—with friends, at parties, and so on—can temporarily boost self-esteem, but ultimately, it can lead to overuse, misuse, and addiction, which further damages your sense of self-worth (Schwartz 2020).

Also, when people engage in compulsive or chaotic substance use, they sometimes engage in behaviors they normally would not, which they later feel bad about. As a way to escape the unpleasant feelings, they may use even more substances, resulting in a cycle they cannot escape. In my experience as a clinical social worker, I have observed that as someone's substance use increases and becomes more chaotic, their self-esteem continues to lower.

Trauma can also impact self-esteem. Experiences of trauma are aligned with symptoms of anxiety and depression. Traumatic experiences can affect our sense of safety and trust in the world, leaving us feeling vulnerable. Experiencing traumatic events combined with substance use can lead to feelings of shame, guilt, and low self-worth. Symptoms such as flashbacks, nightmares, and hypervigilance (heightened alertness) are common, as is harsh self-judgement for experiencing continuing symptoms, which only increases negative feelings and further lowers self-esteem.

Research has shown that improving self-esteem can have a positive impact on recovery. A review of scientific literature for an article in *Medicine (Baltimore)* (Liu et al. 2021) states:

> Previous studies have found that high self-esteem is a protective factor for physical and mental health. High self-esteem can lead to better mental health, while poor self-esteem is associated with a broad range of mental disorders. In contrast, self-esteem is regarded as the core and the consequence of mental health.

When we have strong, healthy self-esteem, we feel more confident and able to make positive changes in our lives. This can lead to a greater sense of motivation and a higher likelihood of successfully making changes in substance use.

Neutralizing Self-Esteem Killers

In early recovery, increasing your self-esteem, or addressing lack of self-esteem, makes a big difference in helping you secure the outcome you want in your recovery journey. And self-esteem is a powerful tool that will not only help you early in your recovery but build on your recovery and have a more fulfilling life.

There are a number of things that we do that can impact our self-esteem negatively. These things could be considered self-sabotaging, and we may not even realize we are doing them. Four common self-esteem killers you might participate in are:

- Comparing yourself to others
- Negative self-talk
- Not living in tune with your values
- Setting unrealistic goals for yourself

Take a few moments to think about how often you do each of these things. How does that look for you? What do you gain from that behavior? And what does it cost you?

Let's look at each of these factors and how you can intervene in them.

Comparing Yourself to Others

The tendency to compare yourself to others is a common issue that affects many people, not only those who use substances or have a history of trauma. If you struggle with social comparison (the process of evaluating oneself relative to another person), it is important to recognize that everyone has unique strengths and weaknesses, rather than focus on what you think you lack. When we look at the world this way, it will allow you to appreciate and build upon your strengths, which can help increase your self-esteem and improve your overall outlook on life.

Social media can also impact self-esteem and exacerbate the tendency to compare yourself to others. Social media often presents an unrealistic and filtered version of people's lives. Social media use can cause feelings of depression and can lead to social isolation and diminished self-esteem. Furthermore, people with a stronger tendency to compare themselves with others are particularly susceptible to the detrimental effects of social media (Andrade et al. 2023).

Comparison is not healthy, and it can lead to feelings of inadequacy. A phrase that has helped me remember this is "Don't judge your insides by someone else's outsides."

Think of a time that you have compared yourself to someone else in a negative way. Think about how it made you feel and if the comparison was helpful. Last, think about how you could reframe your thoughts and think differently in the future. I have put an example in the first row for you.

Who or what was I comparing myself to?	What was the thought?	How did this comparison make me feel?	Was it helpful?	What can I think instead in the future?
Ellen's post on social media about her family trip.	*Her family is so happy and perfect.*	*Sad, because we do not have the funds to travel to another country.*	*No.*	*My family is healing and I am grateful for our Sunday afternoons together.*

Who or what was I comparing myself to?	What was the thought?	How did this comparison make me feel?	Was it helpful?	What can I think instead in the future?

Negative Self-Talk

Negative self-talk refers to a person's inner dialogue or thoughts about themselves when they are self-critical or self-degrading. It's the thoughts that pop into our heads that focus on our insecurities, weaknesses, or mistakes. It can also reflect tendencies we might have to see things in a negative light—including our own abilities and self-worth. This, in turn, can lead to low self-esteem and a lack of confidence. Examples of negative self-talk may include statements such as *I'm not good enough, I always mess things up,* or *I'll never be able to do this.* It can also include harsh self-criticism, self-doubt, and unfavorable comparisons to others.

Negative self-talk can be harmful not just in the ways listed above; it can also affect our recovery from substance use disorder and trauma. Our thoughts and beliefs shape our perception of the world and ourselves. Negative self-talk can affect our thoughts, which affect our mood, which affects our behavior, all of which affect the lens we view the world through. Ultimately, this will affect the life we want for ourselves.

You come to deeply believe what you repeatedly tell yourself, which is why negative self-talk can be so damaging. The more negative self-talk you engage in, the more it will decrease your self-confidence and lower your self-image. If you consistently tell yourself that you are not good enough or will fail, you will start to believe it and inadvertently sabotage your efforts to succeed. And since negative self-talk can increase your stress levels and anxiety, you are increasing your likelihood of returning to use or being stuck in the impact of your trauma. Recognizing and challenging negative self-talk are essential to creating a more positive mindset, which will lead to greater satisfaction in your life.

Some of your patterns of self-talk may be quite long standing. But while you cannot control the thoughts that pop into your head, you can control what you do with them once they are there, and you can make an effort to tell yourself different, more accurate, and more helpful things. Let's take a look at what you can do to decrease your own negative self-talk and replace those thoughts with more positive ones that will help you lead a happier life.

What are some of your common negative thoughts? Take a moment and list some of them below:

_____

_____

_____

_____

_____

_____

_____

_____

Take a moment to really reflect on the statements you have written above. When I was working on my own negative self-talk, I had to ask myself, *Would I be friends with someone who talked to me like this?* My answer, of course, was *No, I would not.* I concluded that if I would not let others talk to me this way, why would I talk to myself like this? It was an epiphany for me. Today, when this happens, I quickly catch myself and reframe the thought. Thought reframing is a skill taught in cognitive behavioral therapy (CBT). It's the process of replacing negative thoughts with more helpful thoughts. It differs from thought replacement in that the thoughts you are reframing are in direct correlation with the original thought.

Now that you have listed some of your own negative thoughts, take a look at them and reframe them into more positive self-messages.

Original Thought	Reframed Thought
Example: *I am so stupid I will never pass this test.*	Example: *I have studied for this test and I am going to do great.*

Another very helpful tool when working on negative self-talk is a CBT exercise called the three C's—*catch* it, *check* it, *change* it. Once you start working on negative self-talk, you will start to notice not only when you do it but when your friends and family do it as well.

One of the first phrases I noticed when I started paying attention to language was when people make mistakes and say "I am so stupid." Taking note of the negative self-talk is the *catching* it. The next step is to *check* that thought. I would ask myself if I was really stupid and challenge the thought that I was. I would think something like, *I would not be able to hold a job if I were stupid.* The last step in this exercise is to *change* the thought, so I might then have thought something like, *I made a mistake, it is not the end of the world, and I will do it differently next time.*

Next time you catch yourself having negative thoughts about yourself, remember the three C's and *catch* it, *check* it, and *change* it. You will start to feel better about yourself and your self-esteem will improve.

Not Living in Tune with Your Values

In recovery, it is important to set goals that align with your values. Knowing your values helps to set those goals and priorities. When you are clear on your values, you can make decisions that align with them, which can help avoid situations that lead to a return to use.

Values also provide individuals with a sense of identity. Sometimes, people who have lived with the impact of trauma and substance use disorder struggle with their identity. They may have defined themselves by how they were, their behaviors, or poor coping skills, and they may not know who they are without those things. Knowing your values can help you redefine your identity.

Take a few moments to think about the things that are important to you. Think about why they are important to you and how they can help you in your recovery. For instance, perhaps a value you hold is "family," and your desire to be present with and be there for your partner or children can sustain you when things get tough. Or perhaps you hold a value of compassion, which will help you to be kind to yourself (when you're suffering or you make a mistake) and to persist.

It can be easy to focus on your weaknesses, but taking time to acknowledge your positive qualities can be a helpful tool in the recovery process. Trauma and compulsive substance use can leave you feeling powerless and helpless, but recognizing your positive qualities can help shift the focus back to your resilience and abilities.

Experiencing trauma and compulsive substance use is difficult. It takes creativity, wisdom, and perseverance to maintain strength while you are actively using. The attributes it takes to not only survive those things but get to the other side of it are extraordinary. Starting the recovery journey is perhaps the most important decision you can make and likely one of your most powerful strengths. Learning to focus on your strengths can not only increase your self-esteem but also help you set and achieve your goals. We often do not know what our strengths are yet when we are starting our recovery journey.

A benefit of understanding your own strengths is that it allows you to focus on what you do best. By identifying your areas of expertise, you can prioritize tasks that align with your strengths, which can improve your productivity and efficiency. Understanding your strengths can help you to develop a clearer sense of your purpose and direction in life. By identifying what you are good at, you can begin to explore how you can use your strengths to make the changes you want. This can be a powerful motivator, as it can inspire you to pursue opportunities that align with your values and passions.

Take a look at the list of strengths below and circle the ones that you have:

Wisdom	Empathy	Positive	Accepting	Smart
Enthusiastic	Forgiveness	Creative	Kind	Assertive
Restraint	Fairness	Spiritual/Faithful	Polite	Disciplined
Sincere	Independent	Modesty	Flexible	Loving
Brave	Open-minded	Candid	Honest	Grateful
Willing	Humble	Funny	Hard working	Love to learn
Common sense	Reliable	Organized	Ambition	Humble

This list is not all inclusive, as we are each unique. What are some other strengths that you possess?

_____ _____

_____ _____

_____ _____

_____ _____

We have talked about what can contribute to low self-esteem and how to combat it. Now let's talk about how to build your self-esteem to improve your recovery.

Setting Realistic Goals for Yourself

There is value in setting goals for things we want to achieve. Goals help us to focus our energy and efforts toward achieving something specific and can provide a sense of direction and purpose in our lives.

Goal setting can become problematic when the goals are unrealistic—when they will take too long to achieve or are more ambitious than you can realistically accomplish. We set ourselves up for failure when we set unrealistic goals. If you continue to set unobtainable goals and you continue to not meet them, you will feel like a failure for not achieving them. In this way, setting unrealistic goals can often lead to disappointment and a decrease in self-esteem.

It's important to set attainable goals that challenge us but are still within our capabilities. By doing so, we can build confidence in our abilities and feel a sense of accomplishment when we reach our goals. It's also important to remember that, in achieving any goal, setbacks and failures can be part of the process and don't define our worth.

So how do you go about setting a realistic goal? A simple system to do this is by setting a SMART goal. Start by identifying what you want to achieve, and then break it down into

specific, **m**easurable, **a**chievable, **r**elevant, and **t**ime-bound steps. This will help you to clarify your goals, create a plan of action, and track your progress. If you want to reach a goal that will take some time to achieve, break it down into small steps.

For example, my daughter wanted to run a marathon. She did not wake up one day and run twenty-six miles. She set many smaller goals before the day of her big run. She started by listening to music as she ran. She would run for one song, then walk for the next song. Soon she worked her way up to three songs while she ran and one song while she walked. And so it went. It took her many months and many smaller goals before she even stepped up to the starting line. Remember to be specific, measurable, achievable, relevant, and time-bound.

One of the most famous SMART goals was made by our thirty-fifth president, John F. Kennedy, during an address to a joint session of Congress on May 25, 1961:

> I believe that this nation should commit itself to achieving the goal, before this decade is out, of landing a man on the Moon and returning him safely to the Earth.

What is a goal that you would like to achieve in the next thirty days? I have added an example so that you get an idea of how to make your own goal.

Specific—*I want to walk more.*

Measurable—*I will walk two times a week for twenty minutes each time.*

Achievable—*Since I am starting out, I'm setting the goal for something I know I can achieve so I can build on that success. I can integrate walking for twenty minutes on Tuesday and Thursday mornings.*

Relevant—*Walking is relevant to my health, which affects my well-being.*

Time-bound—*I'll be walking for at least the next four weeks.*

My SMART goal: I will walk on Tuesday and Thursday mornings for twenty minutes for the next four weeks.

After this goal is accomplished, I can set another goal and increase the time and frequency of my walks. I can't say that I will ever run a marathon like my daughter; but then again, I don't want to compare myself or my success with someone else's.

Now write your own goal.

Specific—_____

_____

_____

Measurable—_____

_____

_____

Achievable—_____

_____

_____

Relevant—_____

_____

_____

Time-bound—_____

_____

_____

My SMART goal: _____

_____

_____

Conclusion

Self-esteem is not something that happens. It takes work and practice. When we stop comparing ourselves to others and end the negative self-talk, we can start feeling better, increasing our self-esteem. Understanding and living our values is another way to improve our sense of self-worth. Last, knowing your strengths and using them to set realistic goals for yourself will increase your self-esteem and help you in your recovery journey.

So, embrace who you are, be kind to yourself, and strive for progress, not perfection.

Chapter 7

Relationships

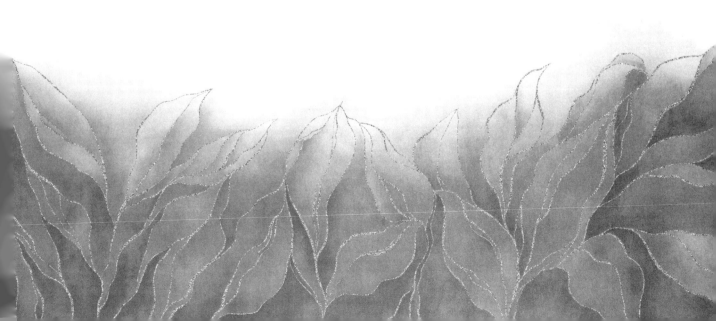

Every relationship is unique to the people in it. The relationship I have with my mother is different from the one that my sister has with our mother. Having strong, healthy, supportive relationships is not only an important but vital aspect of recovery.

Learning to build, maintain, and repair supportive relationships is an important part of recovery. Having healthy relationships and connections provides support, encouragement, and a sense of belonging. In this chapter, we will look at the importance of nurturing those healthy and supportive relationships in recovery. We will also be looking at some tools or skills for building and sustaining those positive connections.

Relationships can be challenging at the best of times. Trauma and substance use disorder can contribute to underdeveloped coping skills, making things even more complicated. However, with some work, it's possible for relationships to not only survive but also thrive during the recovery process. You are likely to even pick up more supportive relationships!

Rebuilding Trust

Part of your recovery may include healing or rebuilding relationships that have been damaged because of your actions at a time in your life when you were not being your best self. When trust is broken, it can take time to rebuild or regain. This is often the case in early recovery. Family, friends, and even coworkers may have many feelings about broken trust. It may take more than saying you are sorry to repair that relationship.

When I think of the word trust, there are several words that come to mind: confidence, dependability, integrity, and reliance. I want my family, friends, and coworkers to know that I am dependable and to have trust in me.

- *My Story*

    Two days before I was to have knee surgery, I met with my supervisor at work to get everything wrapped up before I was to be off for six weeks. My brother, who had been in hospice for some time, was nearing the end of his life. He lived five hours away, and I had not planned on seeing him before my surgery. But as I was talking to my boss, I said, "I have to go see my brother." I postponed the surgery and went to see him. As I walked in the room, my brother said, "I knew you would come."

Only a few months after that, my elderly mother, who lived alone, broke her arm. She told me I did not need to come. I drove the five hours to be with her, as I did not know if she could care for herself. As I entered her house she said, "I knew you would come."

In both of these cases, both my brother and mother knew they could trust me to be there for them. I was reliable, a person of integrity, and they had confidence I would show up. The beauty in both of these stories is that I was not always trustworthy, but I had regained their trust. By being consistent, I showed them I am a woman of my word, and they could count on me even when they did not ask for support. I was able to be with my brother when he died, and I was able to help my mom right after she broke her arm. I showed up. In turn, they also provided me with support when I needed to have someone to lean on. It was, and is, reciprocal.

In some self-help groups, you are asked to make a list of people you have harmed. For this exercise, we want to instead list five important people whom you need to work on rebuilding trust with. The family, friends, and coworkers who are still in your life, or whom you want in your life, that may have lost trust in you due to your past actions. I understand that there may be fewer than five people, and that's okay; there may also be more than five people. It can be overwhelming to look at a long list of people who may no longer have trust in you. Starting with just five people is an achievable goal and it will help it not feel so overwhelming. As the philosopher Lao Tzu said, "The journey of a thousand miles begins with a single step."

List no more than five people below.

1. _____

2. _____

3. _____

4. _____

5. _____

What were the feelings you had as you wrote those names? Shame, embarrassment, sadness? Maybe you just experienced eagerness to work on how you can take actions to rebuild the trust that has been lost. Whatever the feelings or thoughts are, take a moment to write about it.

_____

_____

_____

_____

_____

_____

_____

_____

_____

Although facing these feelings (acknowledging those feelings and accepting what you may have done to break trust) may be difficult, it can often be the first step in mending that relationship. I said earlier that rebuilding trust is more than an apology; it is also about consistency and reliability. We all have heard the saying "Actions speak louder than words." And that is true—consistently demonstrating reliability and accountability over time is important to rebuilding trust. If I had continued my behavior with my family of never being there when they needed me, they would not have *known I would come* when they needed me most. They trusted that I would be there when they needed me most. If I had not created a pattern of showing up when promised, following through on commitments, and just being available when they needed me, they would not have counted on me. Consistency rebuilds our credibility and really shows a commitment to being trustworthy.

Look at the exercise below. I really encourage you to think about your past actions and record them. I also encourage you to let go of the feelings you may have attached to those actions. Look at them as an outside observer if you have to. I don't want you to bombard yourself with negative self-talk, like we talked about in chapter 6. Instead, just look at what you have done in the past, then focus on what you can do in the future.

Person's name	Past example of not being available	What I can do to be present and available from here

It is important to remember that you are not perfect, you may not make all the changes you want all at once, that is okay. If you fall back into old patterns and behaviors, recognize it, forgive yourself, and if needed, acknowledge to your loved ones that you made a mistake and you will try to do better next time. You can also revise your plan of action at any time. It is important that you do not use it as an excuse to beat yourself up. Instead, use it as a learning opportunity and keep going. Change in behavior takes time. Give yourself the gift of time.

When we are working on repairing a relationship, we may feel we are ready to move on, but that does not mean the other person is in the same place at the same time. Rebuilding trust is a gradual process that requires patience and time. Understanding the other person's feelings and respecting their pace can go a long way in rebuilding trust.

Living in the Present and Being Open

When we were experiencing symptoms of our substance use disorder and trauma, we may not have been the best at open, honest communication. If fact, we may have lied, not shared our feelings, or snapped at the ones we care about. We may have also not been open to hearing what others had to say to us when we were using substances, isolating, being standoffish, or inapproachable. Practicing communication skills goes a long way in expressing remorse and seeking forgiveness. Actively listening also helps others feel more connected to you as they share their care, concerns, and feelings.

What are some ways that you have been dishonest in your communication with others? Have you told people you were fine when you were not? What about times when you were angry with someone and did not tell them, but instead let it fester like a bad wound, only to have it blow up later?

Being able to communicate in an open, honest manner takes time. It is not something that is taught in school, although it probably should be. When I was first learning this skill, it was often *after* I had an interaction with someone that I thought, *I wish I had told them what I was really thinking and feeling.* It took time to learn to catch it in the now and to be more authentic in my interactions.

Now that you have an idea on how to rebuild trust and to be open and honest in your communication, let's take a look at supportive relationships.

Supportive Relationships

Having people you can count on and who can count on you is important. Knowing that I have people whom I can count on and whom I enjoy doing things with is an important part of recovery.

I have seen many people enter treatment, and once they leave, they return to use of substances. When I first started working with people who have experienced trauma and have a substance use disorder, I asked myself why they would return to use when they worked so hard to get off of substances. I started looking for patterns in the people who were successful with their recovery goals. What I observed is the people who did not return to substance misuse all had one thing in common. They had people who supported them *and* they had a friend or friends that they could engage in pro-recovery activities with. Pro-recovery activities are those activities that are fun, social, and do not revolve around the use of substances. Let's take a look at what it takes to build that network of support.

Building Supportive Relationships

Creating and maintaining supportive relationships requires effort and intentionality. There are several ways that you can seek out support that is right for you.

One way to build an instant community is to join a formal recovery group. You may want to consider joining a group. You may want to consider if you want to pay to be in a group or if you want to join a group that is free. There are all the twelve-step groups and several groups founded in different faiths, such as Celebrate Recovery, Recovery Dharma,

Jewish Alcoholics, Chemically Dependent Persons, Melati Islami, and others. There are also secular groups such as Smart Recovery, LifeRing, Moderation Management, and many others. You can find a list of groups listed in the resource section in the back of the workbook. Some groups are offered online, and others are in person. You may want to search the internet to find a group that fits your needs.

Many times, I hear people say that they have tried a certain group and it was not for them. As with every organization or group, each one has its own personality. You may find a better match by trying a different group or a different type of group. If you keep an open mind and keep looking, you will surely find one that fits you.

What groups have you tried? _____

_____

_____

What groups are you willing to attend? _____

_____

_____

Joining a group helps you look outside of your existing resources to find new support, but you can and should also take stock of your existing network.

• *My Story, Continued*

Early in my own recovery, acknowledging and listing my support system was an important exercise for me. Each name—from family members who offered their love and support, to friends who encouraged me—represented someone who was an important part of my healing. My therapists helped guide me through the hard emotions I was experiencing and provided me with insights into my behaviors and new skills to cope. Making that list of my support system was more than a listing of names; it was recognizing the people who had or could help me as I walked the path on my recovery journey. Creating this list helped me see that I was not walking this journey on my own. Knowing that I had this network of compassionate people who were willing to help me really helped me get through challenging times.

I think it's important to understand who your supporters are. It can be an amazing experience to see all the people who have or who can support your recovery. Make a list of people who are a support to you. I have listed a few categories below but add more categories and names as you see fit.

Sponsor and or Mentor: _____

_____

Family: _____

_____

_____

Friends: _____

_____

_____

Pastor or spiritual guide: _____

_____

Therapist: _____

_____

Peer Support Worker: _____

_____

Case Manager: _____

_____

Doctor: _____

_____

Others: _____

_____

Now that you have listed those people, what are your thoughts? Is the list longer than you thought it would be? Do you need to work on bringing more people into your life so that you can have more support? Think of a chair with four legs—it is solid and can easily support the person sitting on it. If you remove one leg, it can still support you, but you will need to shift you weight and use your legs to remain on it. When the chair has only two legs, you will need to use your own leg strength and carefully balance yourself to remain on it. You want your support to resemble that four-legged chair: solid with a lot of support.

Maintaining Supportive Relationships

Once you've established supportive relationships, it's important to nurture and maintain them. Having solid relationships takes some work, time, and effort. Below are some things you can do to enhance the relationships you have:

- **Express gratitude:** Regularly acknowledge and express gratitude for the support you receive. This fosters positive feelings and strengthens your relationships. I will often stop in the middle of a conversation and tell someone how grateful I am that they are in my life. This has earned me the nickname "The Gratitude Lady," and I don't mind that one bit.

- **Be reliable:** Build trust by being reliable and consistent in your interactions. Follow through on commitments and be there for others as they are for you. If you tell someone you are going to do something, make sure that you do not back out. Canceling plans or not honoring what you say you are going to do will eventually lead people to stop making plans with you or counting on you.

- **Practice active listening:** Listening attentively to others without interruption or judgment promotes mutual respect and strengthens communication. We so often listen to respond instead of listening to understand. Work on listening to understand.

- **Address conflict constructively:** Conflict may arise in any relationship. Learn healthy ways to address and resolve disagreements, such as respectful communication and compromise. Use "I" statements as much as possible: "When you don't put your coffee cup in the dishwasher, I feel frustrated, because I have asked you to do this in the past." It may feel easier to ignore the conflict, but this can lead to resentment and a "piling up" that ends in blowing up.

- **Celebrate milestones together:** Mark milestones in your recovery journey with those who support you. Celebrating achievements reinforces positive behaviors and strengthens bonds. Remember it's as important for you to celebrate the milestones of your friends in recovery as it is to celebrate your own.

Romantic Partnerships

Many people advise that those new to recovery not enter new romantic relationships for at least a year. There are several reasons why delaying any romantic relationships is generally a good idea. First, the high of early attraction feels great, and it can replace substances and detract from recovery. Recovery often involves addressing underlying emotional issues and developing healthier coping mechanisms. Introducing romantic or sexual relationships early on can complicate this process, as it may be difficult to differentiate between genuine emotional connections and fleeting desires. Often people are not able to see that attraction is not real love. It is not uncommon for people to replace substance with sex early in recovery.

Second, the emotions that are involved in starting, maintaining, and sometimes ending relationships while you are new in recovery can be activating, causing you to return to use, or to backslide on progress. It is hard to work on yourself when your focus is on a new relationship. It can be even more difficult to focus on your healing and growth if you experience the heartbreak of a relationship that you started early in your recovery journey.

Third, building a strong foundation in recovery requires focus and dedication. Introducing sexual relationships too early can divert attention and energy away from essential recovery activities such as therapy, support group participation, and self-reflection. Becoming the person you want to be takes time; give yourself that gift. If you are healed, you are going to be attracted to other healthy people. If you are still having difficulties, you are likely to find yourself with someone else who is also having difficulties.

However, once recovery is more established, it is important to remember that dating is a healthy part of seeing if you will be compatible with someone. Dating is a kind of interview process for you and the person you are seeing. Evaluating a romantic relationship involves considering various aspects that contribute to a fulfilling partnership. Move away from impulsivity and move toward more thought-out connections.

Here are five important aspects of a relationship that a sponsor of mine shared with me years ago. I have shared this with many people and they have found it helpful in evaluating how compatible they are with someone:

- **Mental:** Consider intellectual and mental alignment. Do you enjoy engaging in stimulating conversations, share similar interests, and challenge each other's thinking? Mental compatibility involves being on the same wavelength intellectually and enjoying sharing thoughts with one another.

- **Emotional:** Evaluate how well you connect emotionally. Are you able to empathize with each other's feelings and provide emotional support? Emotional compatibility involves being attuned to each other's needs and being able to communicate openly about your emotions. Are you each able to both give and receive emotional support?

- **Spiritual:** Understand each other's beliefs, values, and practices. Do you share similar spiritual or religious views, or are you respectful and supportive of each other's perspectives? Alignment or mutual respect in this area can enhance harmony and understanding.

- **Money:** Discuss financial habits, goals, and attitudes toward spending and saving. Are you both on the same page about budgeting, debt management, and long-term financial planning? Compatibility in financial matters can reduce conflicts and promote stability.

- **Sex:** Assess your sexual relationship, including desires, preferences, and frequency. Are you both satisfied with your sex life and open to communicating about your needs and boundaries? Sexual compatibility is important for physical intimacy and overall relationship satisfaction.

Evaluating these aspects can help determine how well you and your partner match up and identify areas for growth and improvement in your relationship. When looking at these areas, ask yourself, *What am I bringing to a potential romantic relationship?* Also ask yourself what the other person is bringing to the relationship. Doing this can prevent you from getting caught up in a relationship that is one of convenience, rather than one that you have chosen and is enhancing your recovery.

Take a few moments and consider the five aspects of a relationship listed above. Think about what you want in a partner in each of these areas and then list them below.

Mental: _____

_____

_____

_____

Emotional: _____

_____

_____

_____

_____

Spiritual: _____

_____

_____

_____

_____

Money: _____

_____

_____

_____

_____

Sex: _____

What did you learn from this? Were you surprised? Hopefully, this exercise has helped you identify your thoughts, feelings and values in these five areas. It is also important to understand what your "deal breakers"—those things that you will not tolerate in a relationship—are. For example, I will not allow someone to call me names or scream at me. That would be a deal breaker for me. What are your deal breakers?

For the individual in recovery, it may also be important to tell the people who care about you what your activators and boundaries are. It is just as important for your partner to share their needs with you. Having open, honest communication is the key to honoring each other's needs.

Conclusion

Relationships play an important role in the recovery process, and good communication is key for building and repairing relationships. You've learned about the power of "I" messages, expressing gratitude, active listening without judgment, and being as honest as possible when communicating with family and friends. There's a whole universe of techniques for effective communication that are beyond the scope of this book. For a deeper dive, take a look at *Messages* (by Matt McKay, Martha Davis, and Patrick Fanning), *The Emotional Intelligence Skills Workbook* (by Stephanie Catella and Matt McKay), or *The Assertiveness Workbook* (by Randy Paterson).

Showing up, following through, and communicating openly will help you feel better—*and* help build or rebuild trust. By repairing our past relationships and finding and nurturing new ones, we will not only expand our support network but also increase our chances of sustained recovery.

Chapter 8

Meditation: The Gift of Inner Listening

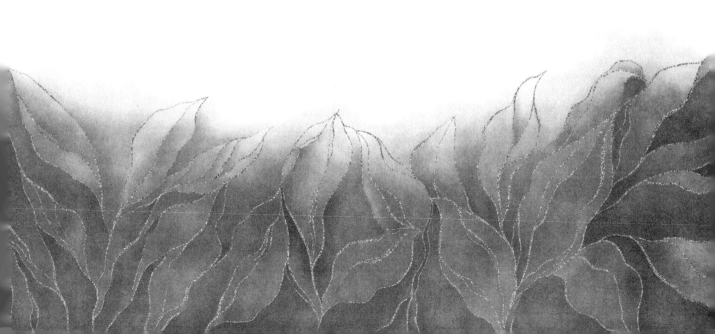

When you hear the word meditation, what comes to mind? If you are someone who has not practiced meditation, you may have a narrow view of what it is. I like to think of meditation as skills, techniques, or practices to help clear the mind. I believe that meditation can be helpful for anyone, including those of us in recovery from trauma and substance use disorder.

• *Katie's Story*

Ever since grade school, Katie had high expectations of herself and always strived to make good grades. After she graduated college, she created a successful career for herself. She started to experience stress and feel pressure about her job and her job performance. This constant pressure for her to not only do her best but be the best started to take its toll on her.

This type of self-pressure is one of the reasons Katie had misused substances in the past. Katie entered recovery three years ago, but she was still experiencing the same level of anxiety that she had when she entered recovery. Katie found it hard to relax. She started to have a lot of self-doubt about her career and even her recovery.

A recovery friend of Katie's suggested that she try meditation to help manage her stress and anxiety. She was not sure that it would work, or even how to start, but after watching a few videos, she decided to give it a try. Katie started with five minutes of meditation daily, focusing on her breath. At first, it was difficult for her to quiet her mind, and those five minutes seemed to last forever! After a few weeks, she noticed a difference. She found herself more present in the moment and not always thinking about what her next task was. She just focused on the task at hand. As a result, she started to feel less stress and pressure and her anxiety also decreased. She not only looked forward to her time to meditate but started to increase her time doing it. This helped her feel calmer and her self-doubt abated. As she had less self-doubt, she felt more confident about her abilities at work. Katie added meditation to her recovery toolkit and continues to practice it to this day.

Many people find meditation to be helpful just as Katie did. Often when I ask people in recovery if they have racing thoughts, they reply that they do. I suggest they give meditation a try. It is very effective in slowing down one's thoughts. Once your thoughts are calm, you become calm.

When the idea of meditation was first introduced to me, it was not something I thought I could do—in fact, I was resistant to it. Sitting quietly for any period of time, without my mind bouncing to what I "should" be doing, seemed impossible. However, with some practice and dedicated time, I am now able to meditate and experience all the benefits of a calm mind.

Meditation may be unfamiliar to some, and maybe you just don't know where to start. Below are several different ways to meditate. Take some time to read them and reflect on them.

Meditation can take many forms, such as:

- **Mindfulness meditation:** Mindfulness meditation is to be thoughtful about the present, remembering to not have a judgement attached to the thought or awareness. For example, "I am cold" versus "I should have worn a sweater because I am cold."

- **Loving-kindness meditation:** This is one I like to use when I am frustrated with a loved one or myself. It is about remembering or cultivating feelings of love and compassion for a person. This can be done by repeating caring, loving, and compassionate phrases. For example, if I am frustrated with a coworker for spending too much time chatting, I might say to myself, *She really cares about the people she works with and wants to make sure they had a nice time off over the weekend.*

- **Guided imagery:** This is the type of meditation I did with my daughter when she was young and could not sleep. I would read peaceful scenes or journeys aloud as a way for her to feel relaxed. There are several of these on YouTube you can choose from.

- **Movement meditation:** These types of meditation include, but are not limited to, yoga and tai chi. This combination of physical movement, mindfulness, and breath awareness can help with relaxation and focus.

- **Mantra meditation:** This type of meditation can be really helpful if you have unwanted thoughts. You choose a word, phrase, or sound and repeat it to *not* focus on unwanted thoughts. One of the mantras that I use if I am fearful about doing something is "Replace the fear with faith." There are several others that I use, such as "I am amazing," "I can do this," and "You are not your past."

- **Body scan meditation:** This is a progressive relaxation technique in which you focus on different parts of the body to release tension, often starting from the head or the toes and moving over the body. I like to do this one right before bed to help me relax. I encourage you to make note of what parts of your body are the tightest. For me, it is always my shoulders.

- **Breath meditation:** This is focused breathing, and there are many different ways to do it. I am a fan of breathing in for the count of three, holding my breath for only a moment, and then breathing out for a count of three. This is really helpful for moments when you are really upset, as it can help calm you.

Of the meditation types listed above, which ones have you tried or are you willing to try? What was that like, or what do you think that might be like, and why?

_____

_____

_____

_____

Given there are so many different types of meditation, how and where you meditate will depend on what type you are going to try and your current situation. For example, I can use the mantra meditation in my car. When I do meditation with yoga, I like to use the space in my basement because it is open and private.

When I practice mindfulness meditation. I like to find a quiet space that I am comfortable in. I prefer to go outside if the weather is nice. I find it helpful if I position my body in a way that is going to be comfortable for at least ten minutes. For some people, this may be longer or shorter, depending on their preference.

Where and what position would you like to be in when you meditate? When considering a location, make sure that it is one that you can access daily. Some people have a designated place at home to meditate daily in, and perhaps a few ideas for additional locations or moments for those less structured meditation sessions, for example, in the car, while washing dishes, or when strong emotions are swirling. Write about your meditation space.

_____

_____

_____

_____

I'd like to suggest that if you would like to try meditation, you start with just a few minutes a day and build off of that. If you start out with a goal to meditate an hour a day, you are likely to give up before you even start. (Remember your SMART goals from chapter 6.) I like to start by focusing on my breath, as I described above: counting in for the count of three, holding the breath for a short time then exhaling for the count of three. Then, I close my eyes and bring my attention to the present moment. As you begin, it's natural for your mind to wander; it's important to observe these thoughts and not judge them. Instead, guide your thoughts back to your breath. Over time, you'll realize that this simple daily practice gets easier.

What frequency and length of time are you willing to start meditating?

_____

_____

Conclusion

The integration of meditation into substance use and trauma recovery is not a new idea. Many people have found that it is a solid tool to add to their recovery toolbox and can accelerate healing. Meditation can benefit you in a number of ways—in fact, meditation practices have been shown to reduce cravings, alleviate symptoms of PTSD, and improve overall well-being (Boyd, Lanius, and McKinnon 2018). These benefits of meditation are particularly notable for those of us in recovery from substance use disorder and trauma, as these are also what we are working toward as part of our recovery.

It is my hope, if you have not tried meditation, that you give it a try. If you have tried meditation and did not care for it, I encourage you to try a different type of meditation. You can adapt or combine meditation practices to make them your own. With some practice, you might find this to be a very helpful tool to add to your toolbox of recovery.

Chapter 9

Gratitude

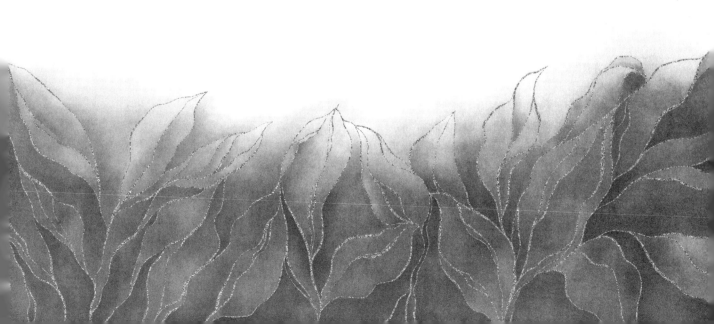

You may be wondering why an entire chapter is dedicated to gratitude. What could be so important about gratitude to take up so much space? Gratitude is one of the best and most powerful tools you can add to your wellness toolbox.

The Benefits of Gratitude

Gratitude plays a major role in a number of kinds of therapy for both substance use disorder and trauma. For example, accelerated experiential dynamic psychotherapy (AEDP), a therapy that helps people overcome trauma and other difficulties such as substance use disorder, uses gratitude as a foundational tool.

Gratitude is a transformational feeling that happens as a result of being thankful for something. Because of this, gratitude has a healing effect. When we care for someone or something, even ourselves, it builds our emotional resilience. By strengthening our emotional resilience, we show care to ourselves, and this changes old ways of thinking and feeling. Gratitude aids in healing from substance use disorder and trauma by helping you break patterns and shift your perspective. One study on the relationship between gratitude and well-being was conducted with three experimental groups, with each group required to journal either daily or weekly (Sansone and Sansone 2010). The first group was instructed to write about negative events in their lives, the second group about things they were grateful for, and the third group about neutral life events. The results consistently showed that the group writing about gratitude had higher levels of well-being compared to the other two groups. We all like to feel our best, and gratitude is one way to do that.

- *Abby's Story*

  Middle aged and recently divorced, Abby found herself living on her own for the first time in her life. Abby had an active substance use disorder and experienced many symptoms of compounded trauma. She felt stuck and overall was dissatisfied with her life. She decided to try something new, so she and a friend took a class, and one of the topics was gratitude. Abby and her friend started sharing daily things they were grateful for. As time went by and the women developed their gratitude muscle, they would catch themselves before they would voice negative thoughts, including gossip, and would instead share what they were grateful for about the person. Abby would even share with her friend things she was grateful for that had yet to happen, saying, "I am grateful I am going to get that promotion at work." The more she worked on expressing gratitude, the more it seemed good things manifested for her. Over time, Abby's life improved in a number of ways. She found she was satisfied with her work, and her spirits lifted. She also stopped drinking, and she credits gratitude as one of the tools that helped her make these changes.

Abby's road to recovery did not happen overnight, but it did start with practicing gratitude. She actively worked to focus on positive things, and thus they seemed to multiply for her.

Some people are more prone to focus on the positive instead of the negative. In the exercise below, let's look at your openness to experience what you are thankful for.

How Prone Are You to Experience Gratitude in Your Daily Life?

In this exercise, you will be able to assess your tendency to experience gratitude in your daily life. Use the following scale to answer each question, and write your answer in the line provided.

1	2	3	4	5
Strongly Agree	Disagree	Neutral	Agree	Strongly Agree

Expressing gratitude allows me to acknowledge and appreciate the good things that come my way. _____

If I listed all the things I felt grateful for, it would be a very long list. _____

Gratitude is a powerful practice that can enhance my overall well-being. _____

Gratitude encourages me to live in the present and enjoy everyday moments. _____

I am grateful for things in my past that have brought me to this point in my life.   _____

Practicing gratitude helps me maintain a more optimistic outlook on life.   _____

Cultivating a grateful mindset helps me focus on the positive aspects of my life.   _____

Recognizing and acknowledging the things I am grateful for bring a sense of contentment to my life.   _____

Gratitude fosters empathy and connection with others, as I appreciate the increase in empathy and connection in my life.   _____

I have an abundance of things to be grateful for in my life.   _____

Scoring:

Add up all the numbers to get your total: _____

This is an interesting exercise to revisit from time to time to see if your gratitude number increases. Gratitude is the attitude that gives you the highest score in the game of life!

You may already be someone who is able to recognize things in your life that you are grateful for. Those of you for whom this is not the case, do not worry. Strengthening your "gratitude muscle" can take practice. The previous exercise gives you an idea of where you are starting from.

Imagine a pile of sand. Now imagine dropping a marble on the very top of the sand and watching it roll down. If you do this again and again, that path that the marble travels gets deeper and deeper. The same thing happens with our thoughts. The more often we focus on what is not going right in our lives, the more often we see those things; and the more we focus on what is going right in our lives, the more we see it. Have you ever gotten a new car and suddenly started seeing a lot of other cars of the same make or color? Do you think that those cars just suddenly appeared? No, it is just that you are now focusing on that type of car.

Gratitude is an emotion that is similar to appreciation, and it is often characterized by a sense of happiness and thankfulness. This feeling of gratitude can be directed toward other people, events, or even aspects of our own lives. To practice is to carry out or perform something habitually or regularly. So "practicing gratitude" means to perform appreciation. It is the intentional cultivation of a sense of thankfulness and appreciation for the good things in life. Practicing gratitude has been shown to have a number of positive effects, including:

- Improved mental health
- Healthier lives
- Improved immunity
- Can lessen pain
- Can ease depression
- Increased energy
- Improved self-esteem and a more positive self-image
- Less likely to judge others
- Increased happiness
- Reduced stress
- Improved resilience
- More likely to make progress on personal goals
- Higher job satisfaction
- Increased motivation and productivity
- Improved sleep
- More generous
- Improved mood

- Increased empathy
- Reduced aggression and less likely to become angered
- Less likely to be activated
- People are attracted to positive people, and positive people are grateful people
- Make you feel more optimistic
- Better relationships with family, friends, and coworkers
- A greater sense of purpose and meaning in life

That is a lot of reasons to practice gratitude! By cultivating a sense of gratitude in our lives, we can learn to appreciate the good things around us and find greater meaning and fulfillment in our daily experiences. Changing the way we see the world changes the way we feel about it and the way we interact with it. Grateful people are happier people. Happier people have a more fulfilled life.

Often in my work with people, when I suggest practicing gratitude, I am met with "I will try to do that." My reply is always the same. I set an ink pen down in front of them and say, "Try to pick that up." After they pick up the ink pen, I say, "Did you try to pick up the pen, or did you just pick it up?" You have to do it, to make it work. A pro tennis star does not just wake up one day to find she is incredible at tennis. It takes practice. The same is true of practicing gratitude; you have to work at it to get the benefits of the practice.

Gratitude List

The practice of writing down as many things as possible that you are grateful for is referred to as a "gratitude list." It involves taking some time to reflect on the things you are thankful for in your life and writing them down. This practice can be a powerful tool and can be used as part of a daily mindfulness routine or as a way to shift your focus toward the positive during challenging times. For this particular exercise, I want you to set a timer for ten minutes, and write as many things as you can think of that you are grateful for. You can use the space in this workbook, a separate sheet of paper, or a downloadable page to write on at the website for this book, http://www.newharbinger.com/54803.

Gratitude

What was that like?

Did you find you had more things to be grateful for than you thought, or was it difficult?

When you first get started, there may be times that you cannot think of anything to be grateful for. An excellent way to start is to think about the things that are a given in your life. Do you have food, shelter, clothes? Can you hear and see? If you lack one or more of these things, what do you have? Take time to notice what's around you. Is the sky really blue today? Is there rain that is watering everything and giving us drinking water? Can you smell the flowers of spring or see the colors of fall? You do not have to "own" things you are grateful for.

The Body and Gratitude

I want to geek out for a moment and explain how practicing gratitude works in your brain and body. I have tried to make this as simple as I can. I find it intriguing, and yet I do not want to get too technical in my description.

The part of the brain that is most affected by practicing gratitude is in the frontal lobe. This area of the brain is responsible for many things. One section deals with such things as how we process rewards, decision making, and emotional regulation. It is activated when we experience positive emotions, such as gratitude. This area of the brain is also associated with empathy, social cognition, and moral reasoning. By practicing gratitude, we can strengthen the pathway related to positive thinking and emotional regulation, which can lead to greater empathy and understanding of others (Sansone and Sansone 2010).

Serotonin is a chemical in our brains and bodies that helps regulate functions such as mood, appetite, and sleep. Having low levels of serotonin is linked to depression and anxiety. Gratitude increases the amount of serotonin our bodies make, which makes us feel good and happy. (Fun fact: Most people think serotonin is produced in the brain, but the truth is most of the serotonin our bodies make is produced in the intestines.)

Dopamine is another chemical our bodies produce that helps us regulate movement, mood, attention, and reward-motivated behavior. It is made naturally in the body and is linked with feelings of pleasure. Practicing gratitude can reduce symptoms of depression (Oppland 2017)

• *Dee's Story*

Dee's substance use disorder started at a very young age. She entered recovery as a teen, but in her thirties had a return of use. Dee had never addressed her trauma, which left her feeling alone, isolated, and depressed much of the time. She was filled with shame that she could not regain her recovery, which had once come so easily for her. She focused her thoughts on what she believed she had done wrong and how her life was such a failure, which made her feel worse.

One day, Dee met a woman who told her to "practice gratitude." Dee did not think that it would help, but she was so overwhelmed by her emotions, she decided to give it a try. She started by agreeing to text the woman three things she was grateful for every day. In the beginning, because Dee felt so bad, this was difficult for her. So she started with very simple "gratefuls." She was grateful for her apartment, her job that provided money, and her cat. Gradually, as Dee shared these things, she started to feel better and she started writing down what she was grateful for. Then she began telling her family that she was grateful for them. Dee found that not only was she able to abstain from substances but the trauma that she had previously never acknowledged was easier to examine—she could see how it affected the way she reacted to situations. Her depression lifted and she once again was active in her recovery community.

Dee's story demonstrates the benefits that practicing gratitude can bring into one's life. When you sit in negative thoughts, that is what manifests, seemingly compounding problems. However, when you focus on what is good in your life and what you are thankful for, your life brightens, and you have more energy to bring even more of that good into your life. For Dee, actively working on what she was grateful for decreased her symptoms of depression, which helped her feel better overall.

Now that you have a little knowledge of how and why our bodies respond so well to practicing gratitude, let's learn about one of the most important types of gratitude—gratitude for ourselves.

Self-Gratitude

When we express gratitude toward ourselves, we are essentially practicing self-love. Self-love is important for several reasons. It helps to build a positive self-image and improve self-esteem. We are more likely to care for our physical and mental health when we love ourselves. We can better set healthy boundaries and make choices that align with our values and goals. Gratitude for self leads to greater resilience and emotional stability as we become more self-aware and better equipped to handle life's challenges. Finally, self-love can improve our relationships with others as we become more accepting and compassionate toward ourselves and, in turn, toward others.

For this exercise, find a quiet, comfortable place. Take a deep breath in and hold it for the count of three. As you exhale, think to yourself the phrase *I am grateful for me*. In the space below, write down all the things you are grateful for about yourself. Give yourself as much time as you need. It is okay to pause and think about all the parts of yourself that you are thankful for.

_____

_____

_____

_____

_____

_____

_____

_____

_____

You have been given a few opportunities to practice some gratitude exercises, but there are so many more that you may find helpful. Below are ten different activities you can try to help you make practicing gratitude part of your daily routine. There are a number of ways you can do this; it is important that you try all of them until you find the one that fits you.

- **Start your day with gratitude.** One of the best ideas is to start your day with gratitude. I have an elderly friend who says that she is always grateful for at least three things first thing in the morning: "I am grateful when I wake up, sit up, and stand up." She calls them her "up" gratitudes!

- **Share your gratitude for your family and friends with them.** Don't wait for Thanksgiving or Harvest Festival to tell your loved ones you are grateful for them. Tell them today! One of the best ways to stop being angry with someone who has irritated you is to think of all the things you are grateful for about that person.

- **Three new things to be grateful for.** This is my personal favorite of all the gratitude exercises. Think of three things that you are grateful for each day and share them with the people you love. This can be done via text, in the car, or at the dinner table. When sitting down to dinner, ask everyone to share three things they were grateful for that day. This is a great family exercise. I have a friend I text daily with three things I am grateful for, and she will reply with three things she is grateful for.

    The caveat is that you cannot repeat the same thing twice. Ever. There is a reason for no repeats, and it is called *hedonic adaptation*. Have you ever gotten a new outfit that you really loved? How long did it take before that love wore off because you "got used to it"? The same is true when we list what we are grateful for. Over time, after repeated exposure to the same emotion-producing stimulus, we tend to experience less of the emotion. Put more simply, we get used to the good (or bad) things that happen to us. We stop seeing those things we are used to as positives and start taking them for granted or even complaining. So, to stop this from happening, you will need to look for three new things every day to focus on to fight hedonic adaptation and maximize happiness.

- **Spread gratitude via your social media platforms.** Instead of just posting a picture of your family, add the gratitude you feel for them. I often post vacation pictures and add captions like "grateful to be camping with my daughter."

    During the month of November, I post a picture of a different letter each day and ask folks to tell me something they are grateful for that starts with that letter. By the time I am halfway through the alphabet, people are looking forward to my morning post. The letters Q, X, and Z are challenging, so I break the rules and say to post anything you are grateful for on those days.

- **Keep a gratitude journal.** Writing down what you are grateful for is a great way of bringing gratitude into your consciousness. It is also fun to look back at different days to see what it was that you were thankful for. I keep my gratitude journal by my bed. Each night before I go to sleep, I write three things I was grateful for that day. You can write as much or as little as you like. For me, I write only the date and three words. There have been times when I looked back on what I was grateful for last year or even a few years ago. Sometimes I will snap a picture of those entries and send it to the person it was about.

- **Gifts of gratitude.** This can be as elaborate or as simple as you want. Cut paper into small strips. I like to use one-by-three-inch pieces. If you want to use colored paper, that will make the end product prettier. Think of someone you love and write as many things as you can about them that you are grateful for on each strip of paper. Place the papers in a box, jar, or another receptacle and give the "gratefuls" as a gift. For example, the year my sister turned fifty, I used multiple colors of paper and wrote fifty different things I was grateful for about her: her humor, her willingness to help me learn to read as a kid, and so on. I put the papers in a jar and labeled it "Grateful for you." She loved it and it made me feel closer and more appreciative of her.

- **Speed gratitude.** This exercise requires multiple players, so it is great for a family—and kids love it. You get in a circle and take turns saying what you are grateful for. There can be no repeats. If your daughter says she is grateful for her family, you can say that you are grateful for your mom, but no one can say family again; if they do, they are out, and the game continues. You also have to go fast, but not so fast that no one can say what they are grateful for. A good way to keep time is to clap three times, and if they cannot answer by then, they are out. The last person remaining wins. You can offer a small prize if you would like.

- **Gratitude rock.** A rock? This may sound absurd but hang in there with me for a moment. Find a rock or a stone, one that you like, is small, and fits in your hand. Maybe it is pretty or smooth or a nice color, or maybe you like it because you found it in a special spot. You can also use a different small object if you like, such as a token or small amulet. Carry the rock in your pocket, or put it on your desk or another place you will frequently see it. Whenever you see it or touch it, pause and think of at least one thing you are grateful for. Anything you are grateful for will do, including the sun shining, your dog giving you kisses, or family.

If you carry the rock in your pocket or wear it as jewelry, at the end of the day when you take it out of your pocket or off your body, remember all the things you were grateful for that day. When you put it back in your pocket in the morning, pause again and remember all you were grateful for yesterday.

- **Sitting in gratitude.** Wherever you are, stop and look around. As you do, take notice of all the things you are grateful for. When you see a picture of a loved one, remind yourself why you are grateful for them. When you see the desk light on, remember that you are grateful for electricity, and so on.

    If you are having difficulty cultivating things you are grateful for, try these gratitude prompts:

    - *I'm grateful for these three things I hear:*
    - *I'm grateful for these three things I see:*
    - *I'm grateful for these three things I smell:*
    - *I'm grateful for these three things I touch/feel:*
    - *I'm grateful for these three things I taste:*
    - *I'm grateful for these three blue (or another color) things:*
    - *I'm grateful for these three animals/birds:*
    - *I'm grateful for these three friends:*
    - *I'm grateful for these three family members:*
    - *I'm grateful for these three things in my home:*

Conclusion

Gratitude is a powerful and transformative practice that can profoundly impact our lives. We have learned the benefits of this practice and covered a variety of ways to practice gratitude. As you move forward on your recovery from substance use disorder and trauma, it is important to remember the healing effects of gratitude. By regularly acknowledging and appreciating the positive aspects of your life, you cultivate a mindset that attracts more positivity and resilience.

Throughout this chapter, you've learned various techniques to incorporate gratitude into your daily routine. Whether through journaling, expressing thanks to others, or mindful reflection, these practices can help you develop a more grateful heart and mind. Remember that gratitude is a habit that grows stronger with consistent practice. My hope for you is that you gain an understanding that you will gain happiness though a grateful heart.

Chapter 10

Recovery Planning

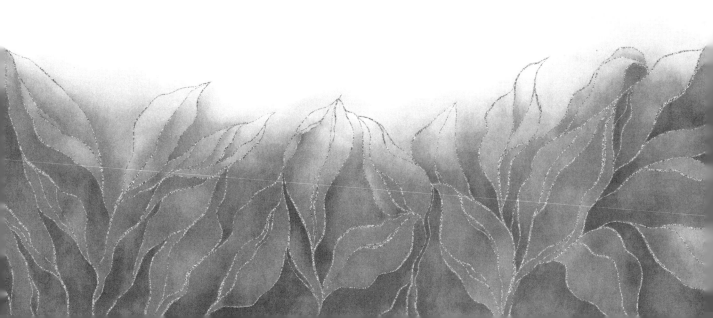

As stated before, recovery is a journey and is unique to you. Often in support groups, treatment programs and self-help books, there is an emphasis on relapse prevention; but remember, abstinence is not a goal of everyone's recovery. If we go back to SAMHSA's (2012) definition of recovery ("a process of change through which individuals improve their health and wellness, live self-directed lives, and strive to reach their full potential"), we are reminded that abstinence is not required for one to be in recovery.

For this reason, I prefer to focus on recovery planning instead of relapse prevention. Relapse prevention is about looking back at what caused you problems in the past. Recovery planning is about looking forward to what you want your life to look like. Life in recovery from substance use disorder and trauma can be incredibly rewarding and fulfilling. Recovery brings a sense of freedom and clarity, as well as the opportunity to pursue passions and goals that may have been neglected. It's a chance to rediscover yourself, form healthier relationships, and embrace a more balanced and purposeful way of life. One of the elements that has made my recovery richer has been forward-focused recovery.

- *My Story*

  I came to recovery at a young age. I had already experienced a number of traumatic events, as is often the case with people with a substance use disorder. Once I completed treatment, I became active in my own recovery. I went to support meetings and made new friends. I went to school and started working in the helping profession.

  Then I slowly stopped doing what had worked for me in the past. I no longer went to meetings and stopped contacting my sponsor. After a number of years in recovery, I returned to substance use.

  Eventually, I realized that that was not the path I wanted to live, and I returned to recovery and started doing again all the things that had worked for me before. For a long time, going to meetings, being with friends, and taking time to relax all worked again, until once again I stopped and returned to using substances.

  It was difficult to return to recovery a third time; but this time, I did not do just the one or two things I listed above that had worked for me in the past. I made a plan—a recovery plan. This was life changing.

It was important for me to look at my past trauma and no longer let it affect me that way it had been. I learned new coping skills and I practiced them daily. I visualized what I wanted my life to look like, I worked hard to get that life, and I am keeping it.

Assessing Your Recovery Capital

An important step in recovery planning is to look at the resources that you have or have access to that will aid in your recovery. All of these resources together are your *recovery capital*.

The term "recovery capital" was first introduced by Granfield and Cloud (1999) in their seminal work on natural recovery from substance use disorders. They defined it as "the breadth and depth of internal and external resources that can be drawn upon to initiate and sustain recovery from substance misuse." Think of recovery capital as everything you have at your disposal to help you in your recovery. We will cover some recovery capital areas below.

Personal Recovery Capital

Personal or *human recovery capital* refers to your resources or skills and knowledge you possess. This type of recovery capital encompasses your physical wellness and how you maintain that wellness. This idea includes regular medical care—making sure that you see your primary care provider and do your annual screening. It also entails eating a diet that is balanced and includes fruits, vegetables, and water. Exercise and adequate sleep are also important factors. One study on recovery capital found that individuals with better physical health have higher rates of sustained recovery (Cloud and Granfield 2008).

Access to mental health services and therapy can bolster human recovery capital. Psychological well-being, resilience, and the ability to manage stress and emotions are vital. Another study that measured outcomes of continued care following substance use disorder treatment found that mental health interventions, such as cognitive-behavioral therapy (CBT), can significantly enhance recovery outcomes (Kelly and White 2011).

Spirituality has been associated with improved coping mechanisms and a higher likelihood of sustained recovery (Leigh, Bowen, and Marlatt 2005). For many, a sense of spirituality or connection to a higher purpose provides strength and motivation. This conviction of life having meaning could be gained through either religious or more personal, nonreligious practices.

The last element of personal recovery capital is self-confidence in your ability to reach your recovery goals. Knowing you have the skills to cope with challenges along the way also increases your success in sustaining the recovery you want.

Social Recovery Capital

Social recovery capital refers to the support available from your social network. Positive, supportive relationships with family, friends, or friends who have become family (this last group, I refer to as "framily") can provide not only emotional support but practical assistance as well. When someone has supportive people involved in their treatment, they tend to have better outcomes than those who do not have support (Bandura 1997). Another way to increase your social recovery capital is to participate in self-help groups like AA, NA, Trauma Anonymous, and others, which offer supportive environments where individuals can share experiences and strategies for recovery. There is a list of some of these in the resource section at the end of this workbook. The connections you create at these groups can connect you with people who not only support your recovery goals but can also can offer companionship, encouragement, and accountability. Additionally, attending recovery-oriented groups can provide a sense of belonging as well as help break down internal stigma.

Community Recovery Capital

Community recovery capital includes the resources available in the wider community, such as availability of quality treatment programs, counseling, and aftercare services. Being able to access these services will fortify your recovery.

Having stable housing that you are comfortable in supports your recovery as well. Stable housing is more than a place that you can call your home—it is also about feeling safe in the neighborhood and whom you live with.

Early in my career, I learned that having a meaningful activity to participate in improves outcomes. Over the years, I have seen this play out for other people, over and over. Clients that I work with who have jobs, school, or volunteer work that they enjoy did much better than those who did not. Having meaningful employment or educational opportunities supports recovery by providing stability and a sense of purpose (Leigh, Bowen, and Marlatt 2005).

Last, sometimes people come to recovery with some legal issues. These might be a driving violation, custody, child support, or divorce, to name a few. Having access to assistance with legal questions and other social services can help you navigate the complexities of these issues and reduce barriers to success (Bandura 1997).

Cultural Recovery Capital

Cultural recovery capital is the values, beliefs, and norms of the broader society that influence recovery. The acceptance of recovery and reduced stigma regarding substance use disorder in your community can create a more supportive environment for those of us in recovery. Stigma reduction campaigns have been shown to improve recovery outcomes by encouraging individuals to seek help and support (Bandura 1997). Also of importance is culturally competent care. Care that is sensitive and tailored to diverse individual needs can increase your recovery capital.

Now it's time for you to think about what you want for your recovery and your life. Take a few moments to think about the next sentence, then write your thoughts down in the space provided:

If you had a magic wand and could create the life you wanted in the next year, what would it look like?

Were there any surprises in your answers, and if so, what were they?

_____

_____

_____

Was there anything that seemed unattainable? If so, is it unattainable, or will it just be hard?

_____

_____

_____

Your Recovery Plan

A comprehensive recovery plan should encompass various areas of life to ensure a well-rounded approach to healing and growth. According to SAMHSA (2023), there are four dimensions of recovery, which encompass various aspects of the healing journey:

- Health
- Home
- Community
- Purpose

We can use these dimensions as a starting point for recovery planning.

Health

Our health recovery capital is our ability to overcome or manage our disease(s) as well as living in a physically and emotionally healthy way. Often when we are in survival mode, whether from substance use, trauma, or both, we neglect our health. Below are some questions that may help you better tune in to what may need some attention (circle yes or no):

Have you gotten a physical in the last year?	Yes	No
Did it include a well-woman or -man exam?	Yes	No
Do you need an eye exam?	Yes	No
Have you been to a dentist in the last six months?	Yes	No
Are you up to date on the vaccines you want?	Yes	No

If you circled no on any of the above questions, what is your plan to get those taken care of and by when?

_____

_____

_____

_____

If you are working with a counselor, therapist, peer support, medication prescriber, or any other professional helper, answer the questions that apply below:

Are you current on your medication checks?	Yes	No
Do you keep your appointments with your counselor or therapist?	Yes	No
If you have a peer support staff, are you keep your appointments with them?	Yes	No

Do you have another provider?   Yes   No

If so, what is their role? _____

Are you following up with them?   Yes   No

Home

Home recovery capital means a stable and safe place to live. Home looks different for everyone. For some, it means living with families or friends. It might mean ensuring a safe home environment by living in transitional housing as part of your recovery. As part of my own journey, I lived in recovery housing while I was in college. This was important to me because I did not think I could live in a dorm where I perceived drinking and drug use taking place. I wanted and needed a space that was free from substances.

No matter where or what you call home, it should be a place that provides stability and safety—not only in its physical location but also in a mental and emotional sense. Trauma can cause one to feel unsafe, even when there is no threat. These feelings take time to overcome. Having a space that you feel safe in is so important to moving your recovery forward.

Here are some questions to get you thinking about your home and if you need to make some changes. Take your time when answering them.

How would you describe your current living situation? _____

_____

_____

Describe if you feel satisfied and content with your living situation.

_____

_____

_____

Is your living space conducive to your recovery and well-being, why or why not?

What are your hopes and goals for your living situation?

If your living situation is less than ideal, what changes are you considering?

When are you planning to make any necessary changes to your living situation, if needed?

Community

Community recovery capital is your relationships and social networks that provide support, friendship, love, and hope. Healthy connections are essential for feeling heard, loved, and included, as discussed in chapter 7. They play a key role in the recovery process, especially when you are having distressing feelings. Instead of isolating us, healthy relationships help to dispel negative thoughts. Rebuilding honest and healthy relationships might be necessary, especially if there was damage to the relationships in the past.

Do you attend a support group, like a twelve-step or other peer-run group?   Yes   No

If yes, how often do you attend? _____

Do you have a formal sponsor or mentor?   Yes   No

If yes, how often do you meet with them? _____

Make a list of any relationships you need to work on rebuilding or repairing.

_____

_____

_____

_____

From the list, pick the one that is most important to you. Do you need to make verbal amends to that person? If you need to change your behavior, what does that look like? What is a small step you can take to work on improving that relationship right now?

_____

_____

_____

_____

Now, write what you can do to improve the other relationships. You do not have to include a timeline, just the action that you are willing to take.

_____
_____
_____
_____
_____
_____
_____
_____
_____
_____

If you have a sponsor, mentor, or therapist, it is ideal to include them in at least this section of your recovery planning, if not all of it.

Purpose

Purpose encompasses meaningful daily activities (such as a job, school, volunteerism, family caretaking, or creative endeavors) and the independence, income, and resources to participate in society. Purpose varies from person to person. Everyone's sense of purpose is shaped by their unique values, experiences, and aspirations. What drives one person and gives their life meaning may not have the same effect on someone else. Therefore, understanding and defining your purpose is important.

Here are just a few questions to get you started on thinking about your purpose:

What gets you excited? _____

What is something you want to explore? _____

What talents come naturally to you? _____

When do you experience your greatest joy? _____

Many of us spend a great deal of time working. Some of us, including myself, find purpose in the work that we do. I spent many years in a job I found frustrating because it offered flexibility. I have come to learn the term "golden handcuffs" refers to a job that has perks—be they financial, benefits, flexibility, or other—that keep you there. Once I took the risk and moved on, I was so much happier in my purpose. I found that releasing myself from those golden handcuffs, although hard, was well worth it. How about you?

Are you in a job you enjoy? Why or why not? _____

If you are not enjoying your work, could you make changes to make it rewarding?

_____

_____

_____

What would it look like if you changed your attitude by practicing gratitude as discussed in chapter 9?

_____

_____

_____

If you are thinking about changing your job, what are you hoping to move toward?

_____

_____

_____

Part of recovery is about discovering what we like to do for fun. Whether it's painting, learning a musical instrument, engaging in exercise or group sports, or exploring the outdoors through hiking, camping, fishing, or gardening, finding new hobbies (or returning to ones we had in the past) can bring a sense of not only fun but also fulfillment. Many of us come to recovery with no hobbies or interests. When I ask people who are new to recovery how they like to spend their free time when they are not at work or actively using substances, they often come up empty.

Did you have a hobby in the past? Is there some hobby or activity that you have an interest in trying? Maybe something that you would just like to learn more about?

Make a list of at least three hobbies or interests you would like to explore or pick up again.

1. _____

2. _____

3. _____

How will you start either researching or trying them? _____

_____

_____

_____

_____

Creating and working on your own recovery plan takes time and effort: time to think about what works for you and even what has not worked for you in the past, and effort to follow through, which is perhaps the hardest step. Taking action and doing the steps require commitment and perseverance.

As you move forward in your recovery journey, continue to refine and adapt your recovery plan. Regularly review your goals and progress—sometimes they change. I find that if I don't review my goals, I no longer pay attention to them. Once I either reach a goal or it is no longer important to me, I set new goals. Don't hesitate to make changes. Stay connected with your support network; this makes seeking help much easier when you need it. My sponsor has all her new sponsees call her daily when she starts working with them so it will be easy for them to call her when they need assistance. Most importantly, be kind and compassionate with yourself; recovery is a journey that requires time, effort, and self-care, and you are worth all those things.

Conclusion

As you reach the end of this workbook, I want you to acknowledge the hard work you have done so far and congratulate you on the journey you have undertaken. Recovery from substance use disorder and trauma is not a one-and-done activity. It is an ongoing process of growth, healing, and self-discovery. But the work, and changes you make now, will help you create the life you want, and more importantly, the life you deserve.

You have identified the people in your life now that are your supporters. Please remember there is still a whole host of people out there that you have not yet met, but who will support you and whom you will support. As the Big Book of Alcoholics Anonymous (2002) says, "We shall be with you in the Fellowship of the Spirit, and you will surely meet some of us as you trudge the Road of Happy Destiny."

Conclusion

Embracing the Journey of Recovery

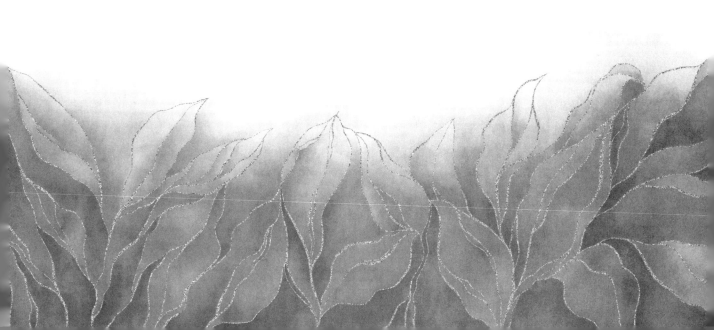

As you read this final chapter, I hope that it not only will remind you of what you have learned but provide encouragement for the future, and highlight that you are not alone in your journey. We reviewed what substance use disorders and trauma are and how they may have impacted you. We looked at the connection between substance use and trauma, and how they are so closely connected: Experiencing trauma increases the rate of substance use disorder, and having a substance use disorder puts you at higher risk for experiencing trauma.

Forgiveness is significant to recovery. It is not about letting someone "off the hook," but about letting yourself be free from the resentment that comes with unforgiveness. In my own recovery journey, many times it was forgiveness that helped me move to my next level of wellness. And by far, the most important person I forgave was myself. If you have not yet forgiven yourself, I encourage you to do so. It is incredibly healing and growth-supporting.

Self-esteem is built not only by doing estimable acts but also by embracing your strengths and ending negative self-talk. Oftentimes, the person who talks the worst about you is yourself, tearing down your self-esteem. You have the power to stop that from happening. Make recognizing your inherent worth and embracing positive self-affirmations part of your daily routine, and the small effort will pay off.

Each person's recovery is unique; what worked for me may not work for you. You may be someone who chooses harm reduction or abstinence, but what is important is that you find your people: the people you connect with and who understand you. Remember that as you grow and change, the people you connect with may also grow and change. Connection to your loved ones as well as your recovery community will enhance your recovery.

Relationships are paramount to recovery. Rebuilding and strengthening relationships and creating a support system are vital to the recovery journey. There is so much to be said for finding people who accept you as you are and encourage you to grow. In my own journey, as I have healed, I have found it helpful to become that supportive person for others. Perhaps you aspire to be supportive to others who have a similar journey to yours, or perhaps you already are that person for others. I have found this fulfilling, and perhaps you will as well.

If you had not done meditation prior to reading this workbook, hopefully, by now you have tried one or two different meditation practices. Quieting the inner critic is sometimes best achieved with meditation. Becoming peaceful is something that takes practice but the payoff of serenity is worth the time and effort.

Gratitude changes everything. It is amazing to me that shifting my focus from what is wrong in my life to what is right in my life has been the key to making me feel good. Life is never perfect; there will be events that are hard and there will be times of sadness, but when I focus on the things I am grateful for, even the darkest of days become a bit brighter.

By completing the work in the chapter on recovery planning, you have created a comprehensive recovery plan equipping you with coping strategies and a roadmap for not just maintaining what you have accomplished but also helping you grow even more.

Every day is an opportunity to grow, to heal, and to move closer to the life you envision for yourself. Hold on to the tools and skills you have learned in this workbook. Believe in yourself, stay connected with your support system, and never lose sight of the incredible progress you have made.

Thank you for allowing this workbook to be a part of your journey. Wishing you strength, peace, and unwavering hope as you move forward.

Acknowledgments

This workbook would not have been possible without all the support and love I have received in my own personal journey of recovery: my family, who have always been my biggest champions—my mama, siblings, and partner have all walked with me on my journey; my friends from the recovery community and my mentors and sponsors over the years have all turned this workbook from possibility into reality. I wish for each of you to find your own community that can be as supportive as mine has been for me.

Last, as someone with some learning challenges, this workbook would not have been possible without my steadfast proofreader, my daughter, Katie. You are a beautiful soul, and I am grateful every day that you are my daughter.

Resources

General

Suicide & Crisis Lifeline

The 988 Lifeline provides 24/7, free and confidential support for people in distress, prevention and crisis resources for you or your loved ones.

Dial or Text 988

SAMHSA

SAMHSA's National Helpline is a free, confidential, 24/7, 365-day-a-year treatment referral and information service (in English and Spanish) for individuals and families facing mental and/or substance use disorders. https://www.samhsa.gov/find-help/national-helpline

1-800-662 HELP (4357)

Harm Reduction

Never Use Alone

877-696-1996

Overdose Prevention Lifeline

Toll-free national overdose prevention, detection, life-saving crisis response and medical intervention services for people who use drugs while alone. Never Use Alone's peer operators are available 24-hours a day, 7 days a week, 365 days a year. No stigma. No judgment. https://neverusealone.com/

Safe Spot

The number one risk factor for fatal overdose is using alone, and we are there for you when others cannot be. We connect people who are using drugs with a trained operator who can call for help in case of overdose. https://safe-spot.me/

1-800-972-0590

Recovery Supports

Alcoholics Anonymous (AA)

Alcoholics Anonymous is a fellowship of people who come together to solve their drinking problem. It doesn't cost anything to attend A.A. meetings. Membership is open to anyone who wants to do something about their drinking problem. A.A.'s primary purpose is to help alcoholics to achieve sobriety. https://www.aa.org/

212-870-3400

Narcotics Anonymous (NA)

Narcotics Anonymous is a global, community-based organization with a multilingual and multicultural membership. https://www.na.org/

1-818-773-9999 x771

Trauma Anonymous

TA is an organization of men and women who share their experiences of strength and hope to help others overcome their past traumas. Their mission is to reach out to those who are still struggling and need the help to break from the bondage of their past. https://traumaanonymous.com/

1-800-893-8800

Cocaine Anonymous (CA)

Cocaine Anonymous is a Fellowship of men and women who share their experience, strength and hope with each other that they may solve their common problem and help others recover from their addiction. https://ca.org/

310-559-5833

Dual Recovery Anonymous

Dual Recovery Anonymous is an independent, nonprofessional, Twelve Step, self-help membership organization for people with emotional or psychiatric illness. https://draonline.org/

Out of the Storm

Out of the Storm (OOTS) is a free and anonymous community suffering from the symptoms of Complex PTSD due to repeated/prolonged relational trauma. https://www.outofthestorm.website/

Refuge Recovery

Refuge Recovery is a peer-led, non-theistic program that uses Buddhist-inspired practices to treat addiction and suffering. The program's philosophy is based on the teachings of Siddhartha Gautama, also known as the Buddha. https://www.refugerecovery.org/

Recovery Dharma

Recovery Dharma is a peer-led movement and community to assist in recovery and find freedom from the suffering of addiction. They use traditional Buddhist teachings, often referred to as the Dharma. https://recoverydharma.org/

Celebrate Recovery

Celebrate Recovery (CR) is a Christian twelve-step program that aims to help people overcome "hurts, hangups, and habits." The program is based on the twelve steps of Alcoholics Anonymous (AA) and eight principles from Jesus's Beatitudes. https://celebraterecovery.com/

Medication-Assisted Recovery Anonymous

Many who suffer with substance use disorder (SUD) have an honest desire to recover but have not felt welcomed at traditional twelve-step recovery meetings or other self-help meetings because they have chosen MAT as part of their personal pathway to recovery. https://www.mara-international.org/

Psychedelics in Recovery

Psychedelics in Recovery is a fellowship of people in twelve-step programs who also have an interest in psychedelics and/or plant medicines as an aid to our recovery. https://www.psychedelicsinrecovery.org/

Harm Reduction Works-HRW

Harm Reduction Works-HRW in response to the need for a harm reduction based alternative to abstinence only self-help/mutual aid groups. This is not in opposition to abstinence only groups. Harm Reduction Works-HRW is for anyone who wants to know more about harm reduction. https://www.hrh413.org/foundationsstart-here-2

Wellbriety Teaching

Wellbriety teachings are based on Indigenous values, spirituality, and community support to help people heal from substance abuse, alcohol, co-occurring disorders, and intergenerational trauma. Wellbriety combines Indigenous values with AA principles and is open to all Native Americans, or anyone who follows their beliefs and cultural practices. https://wellbriety.com/wellbriety-teachings/

Moderation Management

Moderation Management is a behavioral change program and support group for people who are concerned about their drinking and desire to make positive lifestyle changes. It empowers individuals to accept personal responsibility for choosing and maintaining their own path, whether moderation or abstinence. https://moderation.org/

Secular Organizations for Sobriety (SOS)

SOS is not religious or spiritual; its philosophy is based on the disease model of addiction to understand alcohol misuse, alcohol use disorders, and secular alcohol recovery. https://www.sossobriety.org/

References

Abramson, S. 2021. "Substance Use During the Pandemic." *Monitor on Psychology* 52(2): 22. https://www.apa.org/monitor/2021/03/substance-use-pandemic.

Alcoholics Anonymous Big Book, 4th ed. 2002. New York: Alcoholics Anonymous World Services.

American Lung Association. 2025. "Behavioral Health and Tobacco Use." Last updated January 6, 2025. Accessed February 13, 2025. https://www.lung.org/quit-smoking/smoking-facts/impact-of-tobacco-use/behavioral-health-tobacco-use.

American Psychiatric Association. 2013. *Diagnostic and Statistical Manual of Mental Disorders,* 5th ed. 271–2.

American Psychiatric Association. 2022. *Desk Reference to the Diagnostic Criteria from DSM-5 (R).* Arlington, Texas: American Psychiatric Association Publishing. https://www.appi.org/Products/DSM-Library/Desk-Reference-to-the-Diagnostic-Criteria-From-(1).

Andrade, F. C., S. Erwin, K. Burnell, J. Jackson, M. Storch, J. Nicholas, and N. Zucker. 2023. "Intervening on Social Comparisons on Social Media: Electronic Daily Diary Pilot Study." *JMIR Mental Health* 10: e42024.

Arrey, A. E., J. Bilsen, P. Lacor, and R. Deschepper. 2016. "Spirituality/Religiosity: A Cultural and Psychological Resource Among Sub-Saharan African Migrant Women with HIV/AIDS in Belgium." *PLOS One* 11(7): e0159488.

Bandura, A. 1997. *Self-Efficacy: The Exercise of Control*, 1st ed. New York: W.H. Freeman and Company.

Beck, J.G., and S.F. Coffey. 2007. "Assessment and Treatment of PTSD After a Motor Vehicle Collision: Empirical Findings and Clinical Observations." *Professional Psychology: Research and Practice* 38 (6): 629–39.

Boyd, J. E, R. A. Lanius, and M. C. McKinnon. 2018. "Mindfulness-Based Treatments for Posttraumatic Stress Disorder: A Review of the Treatment Literature and Neurobiological Evidence." *Journal of Psychiatry and Neuroscience* 43(1): 7–25.

Caponigro J. P. n.d. "All Religions Practice Forms of Meditation." *Illuminating Creativity* (blog). Accessed February 13, 2025. https://www.johnpaulcaponigro.com/blog/9419/all-religions-practice-forms-of-meditation-meditation-is-a-universal-practice/.

Castillo, J. 2022. "What Is a 'Little t' Trauma?" *A Happier, Healthier You* (blog), New Harbinger Publications. June 15, 2022. https://www.newharbinger.com/blog/self-help/what-is-a-little-t-trauma/.

Center for Health Care Strategies. 2024. "Defining Trauma." Trauma-Informed Care Implementation Resource Center. Accessed January 15, 2025. https://www.traumainformedcare.chcs.org/what-is-trauma/.

Chow, S. 2021. "Meditation Spirituality and Religion." *News-Medical.* Last updated April 13, 2021. Accessed January 15, 2025. https://www.news-medical.net/health/Meditation-Spirituality-and-Religion.aspx.

Cloud, W., and R. Granfield. 2008. "Conceptualizing Recovery Capital: Expansion of a Theoretical Construct." *Substance Use & Misuse* 43: 1971–86.

Early Connections. n.d. "Trauma Informed Care." Missouri Early Care and Education Connections. Accessed January 15, 2025. https://earlyconnections.mo.gov/professionals/trauma-informed-care.

Experience Recovery. 2022. "The Importance of Identifying Addiction Triggers." *Experience Recovery Blog.* October 30, 2024. https://www.experiencerecovery.com/blog/identifying-addiction-triggers/.

Ewing, J. A. 1984. "Detecting Alcoholism. The Cage Questionnaire." *The Journal of the American Medical Association* 252(14): 1905–7.

Feriante, J., and N. S. Sharma. 2023. "Acute and Chronic Mental Health Trauma." Last updated August 2, 2023. StatPearls. Treasure Island, FL: StatPearls Publishing. https://www.ncbi.nlm.nih.gov/books/NBK594231/.

Garbarino, S., P. Lanteri, N. L. Bragazzi, N. Magnavita, and E. Scoditti. 2021. "Role of Sleep Deprivation in Immune-Related Disease Risk and Outcomes." *Communications Biology* 4: 1304.

Granfield, R., and W. Cloud. 1999. *Coming Clean: Overcoming Addiction Without Treatment.* New York: NYU Press.

Harris House. 2023. "Why Starting a Relationship in Early Recovery Is a Bad Idea." *Harris House Blog.* May 31, 2023. Accessed January 15, 2025. https://harrishousestl.org/why-starting-a-relationship-in-early-recovery-is-a-bad-idea/.

Isaiah House. 2024. "The Importance of Sleep in Addiction Recovery." *Isaiah House Blog.* March 22, 2023. Accessed January 15, 2025. https://www.isaiah-house.org/the-importance-of-sleep-in-addiction-recovery/.

Jackson Nakazawa, D. 2024. *The Adverse Childhood Experiences Guided Journal.* Oakland, CA: New Harbinger Publications, Inc.

Kelly, J. F., and W. L. White. 2011. "Recovery Management and the Future of Addiction Treatment and Recovery in the USA." In *Addiction Recovery Management: Theory, Research, and Practice,* edited by J. F. Kelly and W. L. White, 303–16. Totowa, NJ: Humana Press.

Leigh, J., S. Bowen, and G. A. Marlatt. 2005. "Spirituality, Mindfulness and Substance Abuse." *Addictive Behaviors* 30(7): 1335–41.

Liu, Q., M. Jiang, S. Li, and Y. Yang. 2021. "Social Support, Resilience, and Self-Esteem Protect Against Common Mental Health Problems in Early Adolescence: A Nonrecursive Analysis from a Two-Year Longitudinal Study." *Medicine* 100 (4): e24334.

Marschall, A. 2023. "Understanding the Link Between Trauma and Substance Abuse." *verywell mind*. Accessed January 15, 2025. https://www.verywellmind.com/connection-trauma-and-substance-abuse-7269368.

Mayo Clinic. 2022. "Forgiveness: Letting Go of Grudges and Bitterness." Healthy Lifestyle. Accessed January 15, 2025. https://www.mayoclinic.org/healthy-lifestyle/adult-health/in-depth/forgiveness/art-20047692#:~:text=Forgiveness%20brings%20a%20kind%20of,cause%20anger%2C%20sadness%20and%20confusion.

Mayo Clinic. 2023. "Meditation: A Simple, Fast Way to Reduce Stress." Accessed February 13, 2025. https://www.mayoclinic.org/tests-procedures/meditation/in-depth/meditation/art-20045858.

Miller, D. J. 2001. *Addictions and Trauma Recovery: Healing the Body, Mind & Spirit*. New York: W. W. Norton & Company.

National Heart, Lung, and Blood Institute. 2022. "How Sleep Affects Your Health." Last updated June 15, 2022. Accessed February 13, 2025. https://www.nhlbi.nih.gov/health/sleep-deprivation/health-effects#:~:text=Studies%20also%20show%20that%20sleep,lower%20grades%20and%20feel%20stressed.

National Institute of Mental Health. 2024. "Coping with Traumatic Events." Health Topics. Last reviewed May 2024. Accessed January 15, 2025. https://www.nimh.nih.gov/health/topics/coping-with-traumatic-events.

National Institute on Drug Abuse. 2018. "Understanding Drug Use and Addiction DrugFacts." DrugFacts. Last modified June 2018. Accessed January 15, 2025. https://nida.nih.gov/publications/drugfacts/understanding-drug-use-addiction.

National Institute on Drug Abuse. 2020. *Common Comorbidities with Substance Use Disorders Research Report*. Bethesda, MD: National Institute on Drug Abuse.

Nickle, D. 2019. "We Are All Recovering from Something." She Recovers Foundation. Accessed January 15, 2025. https://sherecovers.org/we-are-all-recovering-from-something/.

Oppland, M. 2017. "13 Most Popular Gratitude Exercises & Activities." *Positive Psychology* (blog). April 28, 2017. Accessed January 15, 2025. https://positivepsychology.com/team/mike-oppland/.

Ouimette, P., E. Goodwin, and P. Brown. 2006. "Health and Well Being of Substance Use Disorder Patients with and Without Posttraumatic Stress Disorder." *Addictive Behaviors* 31 (8): 1415–23.

Puff, R. 2013. "An Overview of Meditation: Its Origins and Traditions." *Psychology Today* (blog). Accessed January 15, 2025. https://www.psychologytoday.com/us/blog/meditation-modern-life/201307/overview-meditation-its-origins-and-traditions.

Reinert, K. 2021. "The Influence of Forgiveness on Health and Healing." *Journal of Family Research and Practice* 1(1): 87–97.

Sansone, R. A., and L. A. Sansone. 2010. "Gratitude and Well Being: The Benefits of Appreciation." *Psychiatry (Edgmont)* 7(11): 18–22.

Schwartz, K. 2020. "How to Build and Improve Self-Esteem During Addiction Recovery." *Addiction Recovery Blog*, Granite Mountain Behavioral Healthcare. March 18, 2020. https://granitemountainbhc.com/blog/improving-your-self-esteem-during-addiction-recovery/.

Substance Abuse and Mental Health Services Administration. 2012. "SAMHSA's Working Definition of Recovery." Brochure published February 2012. https://store.samhsa.gov/sites/default/files/pep12-recdef.pdf.

Substance Abuse and Mental Health Services Administration. 2023. "Recovery from Substance Use and Mental Health Problems Among Adults in the United States." Report published September 2023. https://library.samhsa.gov/product/recovery-substance-use-and-mental-health-problems-among-adults-united-states/pep23-10-00.

Tanz, L. J., A. T. Dinwiddie, S. Snodgrass, J. O'Donnell, C. L. Mattson, and N. L. Davis. 2022. "A Qualitative Assessment of Circumstances Surrounding Drug Overdose Deaths During Early Stages of the COVID-19 Pandemic." *SUDORS Data Brief*, Number 2. U.S. Centers for Disease Control and Prevention. https://www.cdc.gov/overdose-prevention/media/pdfs/sudors-data-brief-2.pdf.

U.S. Centers for Disease Control and Prevention. 2024. "About Adverse Childhood Experiences." Last modified October 8, 2024. Accessed February 13, 2025. https://www.cdc.gov/aces/about/index.html.

Volkow, N., and T. K. Li. 2005. "The Neuroscience of Addiction." *Nature Neuroscience* 8(11): 1429–30.

Volkow, N., and M. Morales. 2015. "The Brain on Drugs: From Reward to Addiction." *Cell* 162(4): 712–25.

Wisconsin Department of Health Services. 2024. "Resilient Wisconsin." Wisconsin Department of Health Services, Prevention and Healthy Living. Last updated December 30, 2024. Accessed January 15, 2025. https://dhs.wisconsin.gov/resilient/trauma-toxic-stress.htm.

World Health Organization. n.d. "Social Determinants of Health." World Health Organization, Health Topics. Accessed January 15, 2025. https://www.who.int/health-topics/social-determinants-of-health#tab=tab_1.

World Population Review. 2024. "Cigarette Prices by State 2024." Infographic. Accessed January 15, 2025. https://worldpopulationreview.com/state-rankings/cigarette-prices-by-state.

Yogi Lightbulb Ideas. n.d. "Meditation for Beginners: Simple Practices for a Quieter Minds." https://lb-ideas.com/meditation-for-beginners-simple-practices-for-a-quieter-minds/.

Darla Belflower, LCSW, has worked in leadership in the substance use disorder and behavioral health fields for more than three decades. She has a passion for teaching others what she has learned in those years, and keeps up to date on current best practices. She is vice chair of the Kansas City Recovery Coalition, and is a member of The Missouri State Behavioral Health Councils Culture, Equity, Diversity, and Inclusion (CEDI) Committee. She is also a member of the Missouri State Advisory Council for mental health and substance use disorders.

Belflower is a clinically licensed social worker in both Missouri and Kansas, licensed addiction counselor in Kansas, certified reciprocal advanced alcohol and drug counselor in Missouri, and trainer and educator of Narcan distribution. She presents at several conference workshops per year.

Foreword writer **Bobbi Jo Reed** is in long-term addiction recovery with more than twenty-five years of continuous sobriety. She is founder and director of Healing House, Inc. in Northeast Kansas City, MO, where she has provided safe transitional housing for more than ten thousand individuals since 2002. She is author of *Beautifully Broken*.

Real change *is* possible

For more than fifty years, New Harbinger has published proven-effective self-help books and pioneering workbooks to help readers of all ages and backgrounds improve mental health and well-being, and achieve lasting personal growth. In addition, our spirituality books offer profound guidance for deepening awareness and cultivating healing, self-discovery, and fulfillment.

Founded by psychologist Matthew McKay and Patrick Fanning, New Harbinger is proud to be an independent, employee-owned company. Our books reflect our core values of integrity, innovation, commitment, sustainability, compassion, and trust. Written by leaders in the field and recommended by therapists worldwide, New Harbinger books are practical, accessible, and provide real tools for real change.

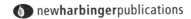

MORE BOOKS from NEW HARBINGER PUBLICATIONS

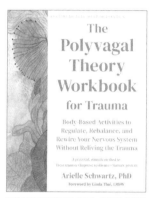

THE POLYVAGAL THEORY WORKBOOK FOR TRAUMA

Body-Based Activities to Regulate, Rebalance, and Rewire Your Nervous System Without Reliving the Trauma

978-1648484162 / US $25.95

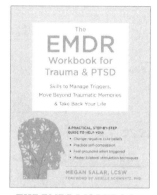

THE EMDR WORKBOOK FOR TRAUMA AND PTSD

Skills to Manage Triggers, Move Beyond Traumatic Memories, and Take Back Your Life

978-1684039586 / US $24.95

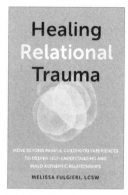

HEALING RELATIONAL TRAUMA

Move Beyond Painful Childhood Experiences to Deepen Self-Understanding and Build Authentic Relationships

978-1648484384 / US $19.95

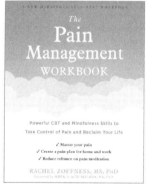

THE PAIN MANAGEMENT WORKBOOK

Powerful CBT and Mindfulness Skills to Take Control of Pain and Reclaim Your Life

978-1684036448 / US $24.95

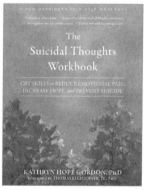

THE SUICIDAL THOUGHTS WORKBOOK

CBT Skills to Reduce Emotional Pain, Increase Hope, and Prevent Suicide

978-1684037025 / US $21.95

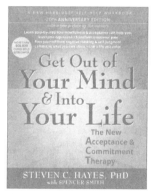

GET OUT OF YOUR MIND AND INTO YOUR LIFE

The New Acceptance and Commitment Therapy

978-1648487750 / US $24.95

newharbingerpublications

1-800-748-6273 / newharbinger.com

(VISA, MC, AMEX / prices subject to change without notice)

Follow Us

Don't miss out on new books from New Harbinger.
Subscribe to our email list at **newharbinger.com/subscribe**

Did you know there are **free tools** you can download for this book?

Free tools are things like **worksheets**, **guided meditation exercises**, and **more** that will help you get the most out of your book.

You can download free tools for this book—whether you bought or borrowed it, in any format, from any source—from the New Harbinger website. All you need is a NewHarbinger.com account. Just use the URL provided in this book to view the free tools that are available for it. Then, click on the "download" button for the free tool you want, and follow the prompts that appear to log in to your NewHarbinger.com account and download the material.

You can also save the free tools for this book to your **Free Tools Library** so you can access them again anytime, just by logging in to your account! Just look for this button on the book's free tools page.

+ Save this to my free tools library

If you need help accessing or downloading free tools, visit **newharbinger.com/faq** or contact us at **customerservice@newharbinger.com**.